# HOMEOPATHY

## *for Nurses*

FOR NURSES BY NURSES

# HOMEOPATHY

## *for Nurses*

*by Maryann Ivons RN, ND*

BANDIDO
BOOKS

Although the author and publisher have exhaustively researched numerous sources to ensure the accuracy and completeness of the information contained in this book, we assume no responsibility for errors, inaccuracies, omissions or any other inconsistency herein.

Includes references and index. Orlando, Florida 2004

ISBN 1-929693-26-5

Cover art direction by David Morales.
Printed in Canada.

To learn more about other alternative therapy titles in the ***For Nurses by Nurse Series*** and to keep abreast of our latest offerings for nursing professionals, please visit us at *www.bandidobooks.com* or contact us via email at *publish@bandidobooks.com* or by postal service at:

Bandido Books
9806 Heaton Court
Orlando, FL 32817

***Nursing at Clinical Speed!***

For order information call our Toll-Free Hotline at 1.877.817.6824 PIN 1174.

## About the Author

Dr. Ivons is a Registered Nurse and Naturopathic Physician. Her experiences include critical care and emergency nursing. She currently has a private practice in Monreo, Washington, in family medicine with a homeopathic specialty.

Dr. Ivons is a former nursing educator and is current adjunct faculty in the naturopathic medicine program at Bastyr University. Her professional ties include *Chairperson for Minor Surgery* for the International Naturopathic Medical Board Tests, the *NPLEX*.

When not practicing naturopathy, teaching or precepting students, she may be found enjoying one of her interests, which include scuba diving, surfing and tennis. Her self-confessed avocation is cooking, especially cooking with stuff from her own garden.

## Acknowledgements

A huge thank-you to Susan. Her technical expertise got this book written in this millennium. To Genie (more then just a secretary), as her name implies, she is magic. Last but not least to the long-suffering, but not silent, Martin. I can see why real authors wax poetic about their editors.

*To my students. I hope they learn half as much from me as I do from them.*

# Table of Contents

**Author's Preface**

**Chapter I: Introduction**

The Best-Kept Secret 1
Theory vs. Practice 2

**Chapter II: Homeopathy a Brief History**

Samuel Hahnemann 5
Symptoms 5
Organizing Symptoms 6
Modern Homeopathy 7

**Chapter III: The Philosophical Basis of Homeopathy**

Vital Force 9
Symptoms: A Disruption in the Vital Force 10
Health 10
Predisposition to Disease 11
Each Person is Unique 11
Disease 12
Miasm 13
Syphilitic Miasm 14
Sycotic Miasm 14
Psoric Miasm 14
Herring's Laws of Cure 14
The Law of Similars 17
Making the Remedies 18
Proving the Remedy 20
The Minimum Dose 20

**Chapter IV: Introduction to the Repertory**

Repertory History 23
Kent's Repertory 24
Rubrics 27
Grading & Assessing Remedies Under Each Rubric 28
Additional Notations & Nuances 29
Using the Repertory 30
Cross-Referencing 31
Choosing Rubrics 31

**Chapter V: Symptoms in Homeopathy**
The Patient's Story 33
Patient Symptoms 34

**Chapter VI: Materia Medica**
Remedy Pictures 39
Common Materia Medicas 40
Materia Medica: Sample Entry 41
Matching Patient Pattern to Remedy 43

**Chapter VII: Case Taking**
Patient Focus 45
Acute Cases and Constitutional Cases 45
Observation 46
Getting Started 47
Chief Complaint and Modalities 48
Causation 48
Review of Systems 49
History and Lifestyle 51
Homeopathic Considerations 51
Organizing the Case 52

**Chapter VIII: Case Studies**
Illustrating the Case 55
Case One 55
Case Two 57
Case Three 61
A Word on Repertory Computer Programs 65

**Chapter IX: Final Word**
Homeopathy for Nurses 67

**Appendices**
Resources
Glossary of Terms
Bibliography
Index

# Author's Preface

Homeopathy is fascinating medical therapy. It was discovered and has long been used in Europe. Homeopathy also has a colorful history in America, where it was quite popular in the early part of the 20$^{th}$ century but fell out of favor with the rise of the medical/pharmaceutical complex. Even though homeopathic practitioners were overwhelmingly Medical Doctors, they were driven out of practice by the medical establishment of the time. Homeopathic medical schools were closed. After that time, Homeopathy went underground. Still, shadows of the homeopathic past can be seen in the United States today. Hahnemann Medical School in Philadelphia was named after the founder of Homeopathy, Dr. Samuel Hahnemann. Today, Homeopathy continues to enjoy a resurgence of interest among both lay people and medical practitioners.

Nurses should know about this discipline for two reasons. First they may practice Homeopathy independently, and secondly, Nurses have patients who use it. This book is not designed to instantly turn you into a Homeopath, but it will familiarize you with its principles and tenets to help you assess if the practice of Homeopathy is for you. Further, it will help you gain a more holistic appreciation and understanding of your patients. It is my hope that this book will stimulate your curiosity and inspire you to want to know more about this exciting medical modality.

# *Chapter 1*

## Introduction

### The Best-Kept Secret

Homeopathy is the best-kept secret in American Medicine. While it is a powerful medical tool, its practice is virtually unknown and unregulated in the United States. In Europe, and much of the rest of the world, Homeopathy is used both by trained medical personnel, including physicians, registered nurses, and by licensed professional Homeopaths.

Nurses are the natural heirs of the Homeopathic legacy. As a profession, we understand that one must consider the whole person even when treating a specific physical condition. The philosophical basis of Homeopathy will resonate with that of the Nursing profession. The rationale for the practice of Homeopathy will not.

Dr. Samuel Hahnemann, the founder of Homeopathy, was born in Germany in 1755. In 1810 he published his classic work, *Organon of Medicine: The Rational Art of Healing.* At the time, although the physical sciences were making groundbreaking progress, the medical sciences were not. Not much was known about human physiology, and medical treatment was crude at best and destructive at worse. To help put things in perspective, Florence Nightingale would not go on to begin to establish modern nursing through her efforts in the Crimean War until 1854, and penicillin would not be discovered until 1928. Given the current climate, Hahnemann's ideas were revolutionary. However, like most forward thinkers, his colleagues did not appreciate him. It also did not help that he had a certain "self-confidence," and as the Bard would say, "Did not suffer fools gladly." Nevertheless, Hahnemann's legacy continues to this day and the practice of Homeopathy, although not completely understood, prevails undeniably as a healing art.

## Theory vs. Practice

In order to appreciate Homeopathy and get the most out of it, it is best not get hung up on theories created out of an 18$^{th}$ and 19$^{th}$ century understanding of science. The fact of the matter is that we do not understand how Homeopathy works any better than Dr. Hahnemann did, but this does not lessen its effectiveness as a therapeutic tool. We must remember that understanding how something works does not bring it into existence, it simply explains the mechanism of action. As nurses, how many times have we read in our pharmacology books, *mechanism of action unknown?* Such lack of understanding does not make the medicine less effective. What it does tell us is that we do not fully understand the consequences of giving that medication and that there may be actions that we might not anticipate.

Along this line I would like to add a word of caution. Although most books on the subject state that Homeopathy is safe, and without side effects, I do not understand how anyone can know this for sure. The bottom line is that *we do not know how Homeopathy works.* Thus, in the best nursing tradition, I urge the reader to assume nothing.

It seems logical to me that substances that can do so much good could possibly do equal harm if prescribed incorrectly. Unlike **Allopathic** medications, Homeopathic medications are not prescribed in a "this for that" way. Each medication has specific qualities. Homeopathic practitioners fit the presentation of the patient with the properties of the medication. In other words, every case of sinusitis does not require the same medicine, because each patient may present in a different way. This can be very frustrating to the new practitioner. Homeopathy is not cookbook medicine, and if it is practiced that way the practitioner is bound to fail. It takes time and patience, but the rewards are great.

This book is not designed to turn a Nurse into an accomplished Homeopath. Such a goal requires more in-depth study and practice. My goal is that, as a healthcare practitioner the information found here will open the reader up to this exciting and sometimes frustrating therapeutic modality. I hope that this book will facilitate a deeper understanding of this fascinating healing tool, and lead to less prejudicial attitudes towards patients who use it. Opportunities for further study in Homeopathy for nurses abound. If, after reading this volume that is your goal, the *Resources Section* will provide a good start.

# Chapter 11

## Homeopathy: A Brief History

### Samuel Hahnemann

Homeopathy was the inspiration of an 18th century German Physician named Samuel Hahnemann. Frustrated with the medical practice of his time, he set about trying to discover a safer, more effective way to heal the sick. In the process he developed the discipline we call Homeopathy.

Philosophically he was very different from the practitioners of his time. He felt that all disease was caused by an imbalance in the **vital force**, that part of us that makes us alive rather then dead. The term Homeopathy is derived from Greek, and means "similarity of feeling." In his classic book, *The Organon of Medicine*, Dr. Hahnemann articulates the four fundamentals of Homeopathy, briefly, as follows:

*I.* The **proving** of substances to be used as medicines, on the healthy.
*II.* The selection and administration of the proved medicines in accordance with the **Law of Similars**.
*III.* The single remedy.
*IV.* The minimum dose.

These four fundamentals will be explored in detail in the coming pages.

### Symptoms

A key principle in Homeopathic thought is the understanding of symptoms. Dr. Hahnemann believed that the body told its tale of distress by the symptoms that it was able to exhibit. He believed that each person exhibited "dis-ease," this imbalance of his vital force, in his or her own unique way. The symptoms that the body generated were the language by which the body expressed its disharmony, and therefore the road map to the **simillimum**, the similar remedy needed to cure the patient by rebalancing the vital force.

Each Homeopathic medicine, has a characteristic set of symptoms arrived at by the proving –more on proving later. Suffice to say, that after a few hundred substances were "proven" there was quite a list of symptoms belonging to the various medications. In addition, more than one remedy could have symptoms in common with another and this could be problematic when trying to decide a remedy for a patient. A way to organize symptom sets and remedies had to be developed.

**Organizing Symptoms**

To facilitate the process of remedy selection, two general types of books were developed to help with the organization of symptoms. One is the **Materia Medicas.** Materia Medicas are books that describe the proving of substances that are used as remedies. They contain the name of the remedy and a list of the symptoms elicited from **provers** organized by body part. As the years went on, these books contained not only the provings, but also the clinical observations of many Homeopathic practitioners.

The second general type of Homeopathic reference book is the **Homeopathic Repertory**. These books contain a list of **rubrics** that describe various symptoms that a patient expresses. The books have changed greatly over time, both in content and organization. The idea, however, is to organize symptomatology in an orderly fashion so that it may be accessed efficiently.

Dr. Hahnemann created the first repertory in 1805. This volume was hard to use because it was organized alphabetically. The next big push to organize symptoms was made by Clemens Maria Boenninghausen in 1832. It was organized by **modalities**. Between 1805 and 1877 there were a number or of repertories written. They were organized in many ways, by provings, by modalities, and by clinical presentations. In 1877, Dr. James Tyler Kent, needing a better tool, and unsatisfied with the information available at the time, decided to compile his own repertory. He drew his information primarily form the works of Lee and Lippe, just as they had built on the work of others.

The story of Kent's repertory is a fascinating one but too long for this book. The fact is that this monumental work, *The Repertory of the Homeopathic Materia Medica,* has been the gold standard of modern repertories until very recently. In fact modern repertories are based on and organized like Kent's Repertory. Modern repertories are expanded by new provings and updated clinical information. In succeeding chapters we will explore Kent's repertory in depth and also look at some examples of remedies from Materia Medica.

**Modern Homeopathy**

Homeopathy has now leaped into the computer age. Computer programs are available that have many repertories on them. These programs also do the tedious job of cross-referencing the various remedies under the chosen rubrics. Although these modern miracles may make the whole process less time consuming, the repertorization is only as good as the rubrics the practitioner chooses to use. The machine cannot replace clinical judgment.

Today, Homeopathy is generally viewed as an alternative therapy in American healthcare. As such, it is a growing discipline, with more practitioners and more patients seeking treatment. Currently, the practice of Homeopathy, per se, is not regulated in the United States. Nurses are free to practice this art, as it is not the exclusive domain of any one profession. There are Homeopathic Nurses Associations around the country that can connect nurses with educational opportunities as well as case conferences. You may refer to the back of the book for a list of resources.

# Chapter III

## The Philosophical Basis of Homeopathy

### Vital Force

The nursing profession has always understood the concept of treating the whole person when attempting to help or heal a patient. The concept of vital force should resonate forcefully with the philosophy that nurses have used through the years.

In Hahnemann's day, medicine was primitive, at best, and dangerous at its worst. Medical sciences, like physiology, were in their infancy. Methods of treatment were barbaric and dangerous. Mercury, for example, was used routinely for the treatment of many kinds of infections and other conditions. Bleeding and purging were common practices. There was no organized philosophical basis for the practice of medicine.

Hanhnemann articulated an underlying principal that governed all living things. He called it the vital force and postulated that it was the substance that animated every thing alive in the world. The vital force is the essence of life. A healthy organism was one in which the vital force was in balance. Hahnemann felt that a disruption in the vital force caused disease. When the vital force is balanced, the organism is well. Any imbalance in the vital force sets in motion the disease process. In turn, the disease state can be recognized and evaluated by the symptoms that each individual organism manifests. Those symptoms are a road map that leads us to a remedy that will cure the diseased state by re-balancing the vital force. We learn in Homeopathy how to recognize these patterns of disease through the signposts of the symptoms and to give the remedy or medication that rebalances the vital force and returns the organism to health.

## Symptoms: A Disruption in the Vital Force

In *aphorisms nine* and *eleven* in the *Organon,* Hahnemann explains his thoughts about the nature of living organisms and the role of the vital force in the maintenance of health. He states that the presence of symptoms are an indication of ill health and that we can only understand disease, a disruption in the vital force, by the symptoms that each individual organism presents. It is important to emphasize that when Hahnemann was practicing, knowledge of the medical sciences that we now take for granted; immunology, endocrinology etc., was unavailable. So, in a way, his ideas about disease were correct. There was no way the physicians of his day could understand anything about an illness except through the symptoms that a patient reported, or by observation of the patient and his symptoms.

Hahnemann's interpretation of a patient's symptoms was very different from that of his medical colleagues. Whereas current medical thought of the time was that disease was visited upon the person by a vengeful god, or by mellifluent influences from the ether, it was Hahnemann's belief that disease arose from an inherited imbalance in the vital force (**miasm**), or that the vital force was imbalanced by an external cause acting on the organism (i.e. **exciting cause**). Hahnemann thought that it was the job of the vital force to maintain the integrity of the whole organism. If the organism becomes imbalanced, it is its job of the vital force to reestablish that balance.

## Health

According to Hahnemann, the health of an organism and its ability to stay healthy depend on three things:

*I.* The vitality of the person
*II.* Stresses on the organism from an external source (an example would be, a bad job)
*III.* Predisposing factors, such as genetic abnormalities or inherited weaknesses in some organ system.

We can look at the body of each person as the vessel that holds the vital force. The vitality of the person depends on the type of vessel she is born into and how well it contains the vital force. If we can imagine containers of different sorts trying to carry water, we can visualize how this concept works. A titanium drum does a very good job of holding water and is virtually indestructible. A terracotta pot, on the other hand, holds water just fine but it is somewhat fragile. Not all people's vitality is contained in the same way.

**Predisposition to Disease**

The concept of predisposition to disease is one with which we are familiar. Some people, genetically, are predisposed to have problems in certain areas; whether it is an inherited weakness in some organ system or a serious genetic disease like sickle cell anemia. Because of these predisposing factors, organisms may have a tendency to become ill in the same way every time. So, for instance, a person who gets a head cold and has a problem with their GI tract in general, may also get a stomach ache any time they have anything else wrong with them. They have a predisposition to have gastrointestinal upsets.

**Each Person is Unique**

Homeopathic philosophy, like Nursing, upholds that each person is unique. Therefore, each vital force is unique. Because of this, people get sick in very different ways. Patients exhibit different patterns of illness even though their diagnosis, Allopathically, may be the same. So, in Homeopathic philosophy each person with a bladder infection does not, for instance, get the same medication because the pattern of symptoms for each individual person with a bladder infection is different and therefore must be treated by different medicines. Treatment in Homeopathy as in Nursing is not only patient driven but also patient specific.

## Disease

The concept of disease is defined a bit differently than the general understanding of it in Nursing. Hahnemann described disease as a disruption or imbalance in the vital force. He described three types of disease states: chronic, acute, and the pseudo chronic.

Homeopathically, ***acute disease*** is seen as short-lived, or self-limiting and usually ends in either full recovery or death. The **exciting cause** (the incident that started the disruption in the vital force) of acute disease is usually an outside entity such as an organism like typhoid or small pox.

The symptoms exhibited by the organism are designed to clear the body of the problem and reestablish balance. Sometimes they are so fierce that they may, in the end, kill the organism. This kind of disease always, or at least, generally, requires some sort of medical intervention. Examples of this, in its most benign state, might be a cold or flu where the organism produces a lot of mucus in order to get rid of the virus. At the most serious end of the acute disease spectrum is an anaphylactic reaction, which definitely requires some medical intervention or death will ensue quickly.

According to Allopathic and Nursing traditions, chronic disease applies to long-standing cases where the illness has a recurrent pattern, such as heart disease, asthma, or arthritis. According to Homeopathic philosophy, ***chronic disease*** refers to a lowered vital state in the organism where symptoms last over long periods of time. Because the symptoms are not strong enough to damage the organism, or restore balance to the vital force, the disease lingers. So, the organism lives with relatively low-grade symptoms over a long period of time.

The underlying pattern of weaknesses interacting with the exciting causes and bolstered by the **maintaining causes**, (those life circumstances or habits that continue and abate the imbalance in the vital force) lead to a pattern of symptoms that we call the ***Constitutional State*** of the patient. Hahnemann felt that bodies afflicted with chronic disease became weaker and weaker over time and finally degenerated into death.

***Pseudo-Chronic*** diseases happen when outside causes disrupt the organism, but the removal of the cause alone will allow the organism to get back into a balanced state. For instance, a person who works on the night shift, but who does not sleep well during the day, may complain of fatigue and depression. They go around feeling pretty awful during the day and lack energy. Just getting on a different shift will change that dynamic and the person will feel very well again without any kind of medical intervention.

Hahnemann, like Nightingale, understood that maintaining good vitality depended not only on healthy habits, but also on the environment in which we live. Clean air, clean water, good wholesome food, plenty of sleep and exercise were equally important for maintaining the level of vitality that each organism started with. Nurses are the healthcare practitioners that perhaps understand this best. There is no pill that can maintain good health without maintaining good habits.

### Miasm

Hahnemann believed that chronic disease arose from what he called the miasmatic state. The concept of **miasm** is one of the most interesting, hard to explain and misunderstood concepts in all of Homeopathy. Disease can be categorized by a reflection of their miasmatic state. The miasm is the foundation cause of all disease. It is a predisposition that one is born with. Miasmatic states can also be grafted (just like an apple tree, when you have one kind of apple tree and you graft a different kind onto it) onto an organism at a later date.

Hahnemann described three miasms; **syphilitic, sycotic** and **psoric**. The most serious and deep seated of these misaims is the syphilitic miasm.

## Syphilitic Miasm

The *syphilitic miasm* is characterized by ulceration, destruction of tissue and distortion of function. Diseases that fall into this category are conditions like ulcerative colitis, cancers of the bone, and some autoimmune diseases such as systemic lupus. On the emotional plane there is depression and suicide.

## Sycotic Miasm

The *sycotic miasm* manifests as excess. Manic /depressive states appear on the mental and emotional planes, and the physical plane is ripe with exuberant overgrowths. An example of this would be fig warts.

## Psoric Miasm

The *psoric state* is the most benign miasmatic state. Physically one sees rashes and itching. Mentally, people needing psoric remedies are slow and plodding. They have a lot of fears and anxieties. The world could be a scary, uncertain place for those with psoric constitutions.

## Herring's Laws of Cure

Disease may arise anywhere in the organism. When we think of disease in the Allopathic model (this term includes Nursing, unfortunately, they are considered guilty by association), we generally categorize them as physical or mental. In this model they are two separate things. The Homeopathic concept is different.

Any organism, to varying degrees, consists of a mental plane, an emotional plane and a physical plane. The deepest level of pathology develops on the mental plane; that is, the most serious diseases arise from the mental plane. More external is the emotional plane, and although disease arising from this plane can be very serious and devastating to the organism it is certainly easier to deal with than diseases arising from the mental plane.

**Planes of an Organism**

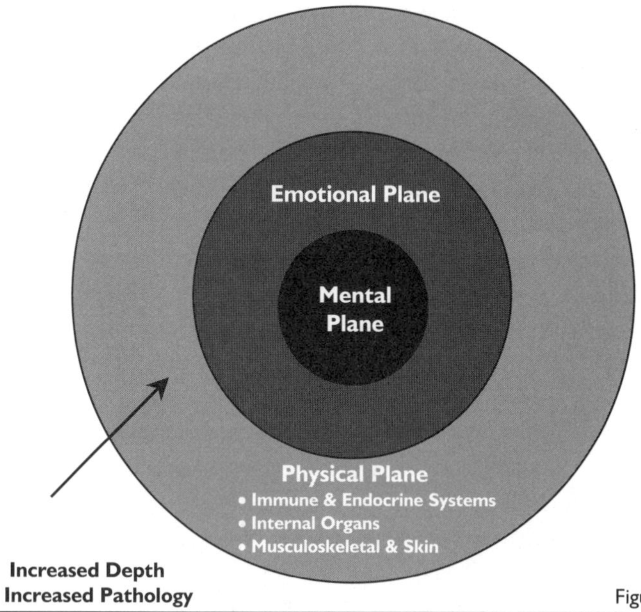


Figure 3:1

The physical plane is the most superficial plane of the organism and diseases arising there are less harmful to the organism in general. The physical plane, of course, has its own hierarchy. Diseases that arise in the immune system or in the endocrine system are far more serious than diseases arising in more external organs, such as the gastrointestinal tract or the skin.

Constantine Herring, a nineteenth century physician, formulated what he termed *The Laws of Cure*. After observing patients for many years, he noticed a pattern of improvement of symptoms, after treatment, which eventually leads to cure. What he described has become a roadmap for Homeopathic practitioners to use when evaluating the effectiveness of the treatment given. When Homeopaths prescribe any medication, they can expect one of four outcomes: nothing apparently happens, suppression of the symptoms, palliation of the symptoms, or cure. Additionally, a patient may experience aggravations. Aggravation is part of the curative process.

The assessment of the effectiveness of our treatment is the criteria by which we decide how to proceed. **Aggravation** is defined as a transient worsening of symptoms, followed by relief. Aggravations and resolution of symptoms will follow Herring's laws of cure. **Cure** is the alleviation of all the symptoms the patient presented with, and no new symptoms arise. **Palliation** is a removal of the complaining symptoms with possibly other symptoms showing up or other complaints not relieved. **Suppression** is disappearance of the symptom the patient complained about, but with an appearance of symptoms of a deeper origin (an example of this would be the disappearance of an eczematous rash, followed by the appearance of asthma).

Hahnemann believed that the vital force acted in an intelligent way to heal the organism. Herring articulated the following principles, to help us to evaluate the effectiveness of the treatment we prescribe for our patients.

Since there is no actual scientific research done on this subject, we would not actually refer to these as "laws." This is just its title. However, if you think about your own Nursing practice and experience with patients, I believe that you will find some truth here. The following is a statement of Herring's *Laws of Cure:*

The direction of cure should be:
**Vital to less vital organs:** If a patient comes in with pneumonia, for example, when the correct remedy is given we would not be surprised to see the rales and cough disappear and upper respiratory symptoms develop.

**From within outwards:** The classic example here is the child who now has asthma after a suppressive treatment of eczema with cortisone. When given the correct Homeopathic medication you expect to see the asthma disappear and the eczema reappear. The eczema will resolve without further treatment.

**From above downward:** For example, a rash that appears on the trunk should disappear from the top of the chest first and down the trunk until it disappears.

**In reverse order of appearance:** This law refers to the progress of the case over time. In a patient with many complaints, we should expect to see the most recent symptoms disappear first and the symptoms of long standing, last.

As mentioned earlier, a word of caution is in order here. Conventional wisdom about Homeopathy claims that these medications "do no harm." It seems illogical, and probably dangerous to assume that a medicine that can have such a profound effect on the patient when prescribed correctly, will not be equally destructive if prescribed incorrectly. If you are going to treat a patient Homeopathically, please follow the conventions of this discipline.

### The Law of Similars

*Similia Similibus Curanture.* This is the law of similars; *like cures like.* Hahnemann postulated that substances that in material doses could cause disease or symptoms, when potentized (which I will explain later) could cure those same symptoms. This, of course, is a concept that is very foreign to us today and not something that can be easily proven. To illustrate, every Nurse is familiar with the use of ipecac for poison ingestion. The action of ipecac causes terrible nausea and vomiting. Homeopathically we use ipecac when a patient presents with terrible nausea that is unrelieved by vomiting.

Whether there is any physiologic truth to this concept remains to be seen. Clinically, however, I do not think it is particularly useful to worry about the lack of "scientific" proof. Having said that, it is important to point out that the discipline of Homeopathy has many years of clinical practice and successes with the medications used.

We have to remind ourselves once again that Hahnemann did not have the scientific expertise that we have today and that his theories of disease were just that, theories. He felt that the medicines that he used produced an artificial disease that was similar to the disease the organism was trying to eliminate and thus, this artificial disease brought the vital force back into balance and caused a curative effect in the organism. This sounds very strange to us today and may or may not be true. The bottom line is that the medications, properly produced, have some effect on the organism. Exactly what that effect is we really do not know or understand at this time. Nurses deal with this sort of conundrum all the time. Again, we have only to look in the *PDR* at the mechanism of action section, the constant refrain is, *mechanism of action unknown*. Thus, what we can say is that Homeopaths seek a medication whose symptom pattern is similar to the symptom pattern elicited by the diseased patient and that this medication is called the **similimum**.

## Making the Remedies

**Potentization** is the process by which substances are made into Homeopathic medications. The process involves serial dilutions and **secussions** of each of the substances in a particular way. The result of this process is a medication that is said to be "potentized."

There are two basic dilutions for potentizing a substance, a one in ten dilution and a one in one hundred dilution. The one in ten dilutions are called *x dilutions*, and the one in one hundred dilutions are called *c dilutions*. The dilutions are made by taking one part of solute and diluting it with nine, or ninety-nine parts of solvent, respectively. The solution is then shaken or secussed.

One part is then taken out of the resulting dilution and re-diluted with either nine or ninety-nine c.c. of solvent, and secussed again. This process is repeated over and over until the desired potency is reached.

The most common potencies we use nowadays are 6c, 30c, 200c, 1M and 10M. The "M" potencies are actually one in one hundred diluted one thousand times, thus the "M" for the Latin for thousand.

*The more dilute the potency, the stronger the medication.* This is counterintuitive to current scientific thought and thus generally, this is a concept that is very hard for Allopathic practitioners to grasp.

Since this concept can be hard to visualize, I have attempted to illustrate it. Consider the following test tubes. One set of tubes is for the 1:10 dilution and one is for the 1:100 dilution, the principle is the same. I will use the 1:100 dilution as my example. As you can see the first tube contains 1 part of solute, the dark stuff at the bottom. Next, 99 parts of solvent is added. These total 100 parts of liquid are shaken vigorously (secussed). The next step is to take 1 part of *this* solution and repeat the process. The number of times one dilutes and seccusses the original dilution determines the eventual potency of the remedy. For example, an original 1:100 dilution, diluted and secussed 30 times would be a 30c potency.

**Potentization of Remedies**

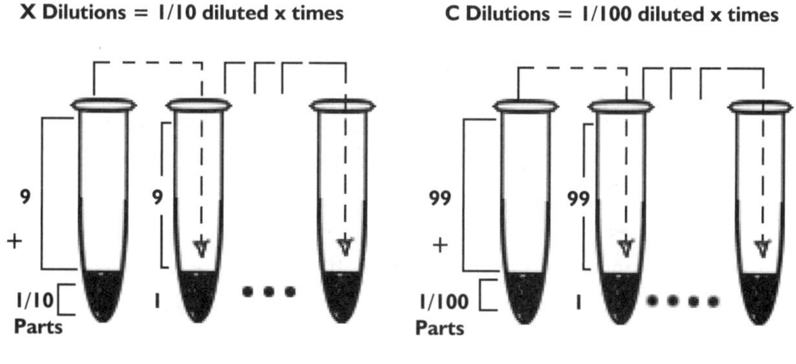


Figure 3:2

**Proving the Remedy**

The concept of proving is an interesting one. Hahnamann needed a way to find out the properties of his remedies. In *aphorism 70*, Hahnemann tells us why and how he will test his medications. He says:

> *"The untuned that we call disease can be changed into health only by a returning of the vital energy through medicines whose curative virtue is nothing, therefore, but their ability to alter health, i.e. to produce symptoms in a characteristic way and these symptoms can best and most clearly be ascertained by provings made on the healthy."*

What Hahnemann meant was that giving these medications to a healthy person would cause a set of symptoms that were characteristic of the healing properties when given to a sick person.

In *provings*, we take a healthy group of individuals, we give them a certain medication over a period of time and when symptoms start to occur, we write down these symptoms and do a statistical analysis of the results. This group of symptoms becomes part of the identity of the remedy being proven. If we see these same symptoms in a person with illness, we can give that medication in order to allay those symptoms. What we know about Homeopathic medications comes from proving and also from clinical results.

**The Minimum Dose**

Minimum dose merely means that you give the smallest dose of the medication necessary and you give it the fewest number of times necessary to begin to alleviate the patient's symptoms. With Homeopathy more is not better. Homeopaths only give medication when it is indicated, and in the least possible dose to give the symptom relief that is wanted.

Although the medications and the rational for the prescription of them are different, the goal of Homeopathic and Nursing treatment are the same. Treat the patient in the safest most effective, and speediest way possible. And above all, do not harm.

# Chapter IV

## Introduction to the Repertory

### Repertory History

Repertories are one of the basic tools of Homeopathic medicine. In the repertories, we find lists of symptoms, called rubrics, which are organized in a very specific way. Under each of these rubrics is listed the remedies that have been found to illicit the symptom described by the rubric.

The term repertory is thought to come from the Latin, *repertus*, which means, "to find." This is an excellent definition, because it is the repertory that helps the Homeopath find and sort the different symptoms that will ultimately lead to a list of remedies that will solve the case.

There are many different repertories organized in very different ways. By 1805, Samuel Hahnemann had proven enough remedies so that the number of symptoms and remedies were a little hard to handle from memory. His first repertory was handwritten, with the symptoms organized alphabetically and the remedies associated with them listed underneath. It was in two parts. The first part was symptoms that he had noted in his clinical practice. Part two were the symptoms he had noted in the provings.

In 1830, Clements Maria Boenninghausen, a follower of Hahnemann, created the very first comprehensive repertory. He called it, *Repertory of Antipsorics*. Over the next fifty years, Boenninghausen refined and improved his repertories. His last book, *The Therapeutic Pocketbook*, is still used today, and it is very helpful in obscure cases.

Of course, no history is terribly interesting without a little conflict, and in Homeopathy, there was a lot of conflict. The first half of the nineteenth century, the followers of

Hahnemann, who were many and varied, had broken down into two basic camps.

The purists thought that only proven symptoms could be used in a repertory to find the correct remedy. Hahnemann had used both proven symptoms and clinical observations when he chose his remedies, but this was not good enough for the purists. In their camp, we find George Jahr, Constantine Herring (of *Herring's Law* fame), and William Gentry. They wrote their repertories strictly from the provings, some of them only using the exact words of the prover. The most famous set of proving references was written by Constantine Herring called, *Herring's Guiding Symptoms*, which were later indexed by Calvin Knerr, his son-in-law, into *The Repertory of Herrings Guiding Symptoms* that was published in 1896.

**Kent's Repertory**

After the 1880's, as the practice and number of practitioners of Homeopathy grew, many small repertories were published. Many of these covered only one organ system, a specific physiological condition, or a disease; for example, diarrhea, gonorrhea, or menopause. All these books were very useful, but there were a whole lot of them. A Homeopath had to carry around many books to practice this type of medicine.

It was during this period that James Tyler Kent, a Homeopath recently of Philadelphia, decided the time had come to develop a more comprehensive, better-organized repertory. Kent and his wife, Clara Louise worked hundreds and hundreds of hours on this repertory. He drew his information primarily from the repertories of Lee and Lippe. When he felt there were errors or unreliable information, he went back and painstakingly checked the provings. This was a tedious and time-consuming process, but in the end, he had a manuscript that he could count on in his practice.

When he was finally done, everybody wanted a copy. However, printing was very expensive in those days and he felt he could not bear that cost alone. He finally settled this problem by selling the repertory by subscription, section by section, over a two-year period, at thirty dollars a copy.

He sold about 200 subscriptions, which generally covered the cost of printing, about $9,000. But, there were more problems. After the first two sections were published, over half of the subscriptions were canceled. Kent did not make any money on the first edition.

Fortunately, Kent did not end up in the poorhouse, nor did he win the lottery. He simply soldiered on. Reviewed, revised, and added onto over the years, Kent's repertory is now the "gold standard" of repertories and is used throughout the world. Modern repertories like *The Synthetic Repertory*, by Barthell and Clunker, *The General Repertory*, by Kuensley, *The Complete Repertory*, by Van Zandvoort, and *Murphy's Homeopathic Medical Repertory* are all basically, Kent.

While Kent is the book most modern Homeopaths learn from, there are some problems with it. The book was written in the early 1800's when culture and the language were very different then they are today. I think we all understand that language reflects the culture and the ways of its time, and Kent's repertory was no exception. You will encounter odd words like "opisthotonos," or involuntary arching of the back. The medical terminology of the 1800's could be quite different from ours today. For example, the term "dropsy" was used for congestive heart failure. These language differences make it hard to find the modern equivalents in Kent's repertory. Luckily, there is a useful guide to help you navigate these rocky shores. *A Dictionary of Homeopathic Medical Terminology*, by Jay Yasgar, is a handy book to have. It can help you translate the medical terms in Kent's repertory into the modern conditions.

Kent's repertory is organized into thirty-one sections, falling into four categories. The categories are generals, anatomy, functions, and discharges. Under generals, we find sections one and two, *Mind* and *Vertigo*. The sections on anatomy, function and discharges are woven together. The organization is as follows.

## Organization of Kent's Repertory

| Generals | Anatomy | Function | Discharges |
|---|---|---|---|
| 1-Mind | | | |
| 2-Vertigo | | | |
| | 3-Head | | |
| | 4-Eye | | |
| | | 5-Vision | |
| | 6-Ear | | |
| | | 7-Hearing | |
| | 8-Nose | | |
| | 9-Face | | |
| | 10-Mouth | | |
| | 11-Teeth | | |
| | 12-Throat and External Throat | | |
| | 13-Stomach | | |
| | 14-Abdomen | | |
| | 15-Rectum | | |
| | | | 16-Stool |
| | 17-Urinary Organs | | |
| | 18-Genitalia and Female Genitalia | | |
| | 19-Larynx and Trachea | | |
| | | 20-Respiration | |
| | | 21-Cough | |
| | | | 22-Expectoration |
| | 23-Chest | | |
| | 24-Back | | |
| | 25-Extremities | | |
| 26-Sleep | | | |
| 27-Chill | | | |
| 28-Fever | | | |
| | | | 29-Perspiration |
| | 30-Skin | | |
| 31-Generalities | | | |

Table 4:1

The first section, *mind*, is probably the most interesting section in the repertory. It not only covers how you feel, but how you think. Speech is covered in the mind section as it relates to the function of speech and not the physical manifestation of speech, which is in the mouth section.

## Rubrics

The rubric is the major unit of the repertory. It is the way symptoms are represented. The best example I can give is that it is much like an index. In an index you have a general category followed by subcategories that further refine what is above it. In the repertory, each section is divided into rubrics in alphabetical order with sub-rubrics underneath. The symptoms are listed in the following order: section, with rubric underneath in alphabetical order; side or part (that is to say right or left); followed by time; followed underneath by modalities; then conditions and modifiers; under that, extensions (anything that starts in a part and goes somewhere else. For instance, pain in the shoulder extending down the back); next locations; followed again by side, time, modalities, conditions, modifiers, extensions, etc. The pattern repeats over and over, and once you get used to this, it is easy to find a rubric in the repertory. The repertory organization would look generally like this:

---

**Using Rubrics**

*Section*
*Rubric* (in alphabetical order)
*Side* (right-left)
*Time*
*Modalities, conditions and modifiers*
*Extensions* (for example; pain that shoots to knee)

*Side* (these are sub-rubrics)
*Time*
*Modalities, etc.*
*Extensions*
*Sensations* (back to sub-rubrics or sub-sub-rubrics)
*Side*

*Modalities, etc*
*Extensions*
*Locations*
*Side...*

Table 4:2

---

What you have is a list of symptoms that is broken down, level by level, to become increasingly more precise. Basically, it is like reading a sentence backwards. For example, say you want to describe a headache that happens in the morning and is worse if you do not eat right away. You would start out with head, go to the rubric headache, time morning, and you would find a sub-rubric: *breakfast is delayed, if.* It would look like this:

---

**Finding Remedies**

*Head* (section)
*Pain* (rubric)
*Morning* (sub-rubrics) etc.
*Breakfast is delayed, if: Calc*

Table 4:3

---

Let us review what we are looking at. I know it can be confusing the first time.

The repertory is an index of symptoms under each of which are listed the Homeopathic remedies that apply to that rubric. We have: Head; pain, morning, breakfast is delayed, if: (this is the rubric). Following that you have: *Calc*. This is the remedy that is associated with this rubric (Calc is short for Calcaria carbonica). This rubric is slightly unusual in that it only contains one remedy. One usually expects to find more than one represented.

### Grading & Assessing Remedies Under Each Rubric

Once you find the rubric, you will notice that underneath it is a list of remedies. These remedies are listed in alphabetical order. You will also note that some of the remedies are in **bold** type, some in *italics* and some in normal type. This method of listing is called *grading*. Grading refers to the frequency with which this rubric, or this symptom, has been seen in provings or in clinical practice, not the vehemence or intensity of the symptom.

I will try to give a simple example. If you have 30 people doing a proving of a remedy and all of them report that they have a headache before a thunderstorm, then that remedy would appear in bold print under that rubric.

If you proved a different remedy and only 15 of the thirty people reported a headache before a thunderstorm it would appear in italics under that same rubric.

If you did a third proving with a third remedy and only 2 people complained of the headache before a thunderstorm then that remedy would be in regular type under that rubric.

Some remedies that are proven, never mention anything about thunderstorms at all. Note that nothing is mentioned about the intensity of the headache. The following is the example of how the rubric would be found in the repertory and the remedies associated with it.

---

**Grading**
Head
Pain
Thunderstorms, before: Bry., lach., *nat-c.* ,**Phos.**, *rhod.,sep., sil.*

Table 4:4

---

You will note that the seven remedies found under this rubric are in alphabetical order. One remedy, **Phos** is in bold print. Four remedies are in *italics,* and two are in regular print. This means that virtually every prover of Phosphorus expressed this symptom. The provers who participated in the provings of *nat-c, rhod, sep. and sil,* expressed this symptom more then half the time. The provers of Bry and lach expressed this symptom occasionally.

### Additional Notations & Nuances

There are also notations and words that are important to understand when using the repertory. An arrow, pointing to the left *(<)*, means "worse than" while pointing to the right *(>)*, means "better from."

"AGG" in the repertory means aggravated by or aggravation from. That is, any of the remedies listed below that are made worse or aggravated by what precedes it. So, for instance, you would have head, headache, heat, Agg (aggravates). This would mean that heat aggravates the headache.

"AMEL" stands for ameliorates, or better from. Thus, the remedies listed below the rubric are better from whatever precedes it. For instance, if you choose: Head, headache, cold applications, Amel; you are describing a headache that is better if you use a cold pack on it. If you see neither Amel nor Agg, know that it always refers to an aggravation.

Another major hurdle to overcome with the use of the repertory is the subtlety of language. Remember that Kent was writing in the early 1800's. Language is different because the meaning of words changes over time. Not only do words change their meaning, they can go out of use altogether and new words can come into use. In addition, there are concepts that we now have that Kent was not familiar with. So, finding the right rubric, particularly in Kent's repertory, sometimes means understanding the language very well and considering a rubric choice very carefully. The subtle differences in concepts are important to understand. For instance, "loathing of life" is very different from "desires death." The *mind section* is particularly troublesome in this way because there are ranges of emotion. For example, there is a difference between jealousy and envy. Anger can go from mere irritability to homicidal rage. All of these entries have different sets of remedies underneath them, and in order to be in the right ballpark when we go to repertorize, you must be very sure about the feelings/emotions that you are repertorizing and that you express them in the most concise way.

## Using the Repertory

Now that we know how the repertory is organized, how do we use it? When "we take the case," we find a list of symptoms that we translate into the language of the repertory (repertorized symptoms). Case taking can be a time consuming proposition and will be described in some length in the next section of this book. Once this is done we choose the rubric under which we will find the remedies that we will cross-reference. This also is a time consuming procedure. In the "old days" hand repertorizing could take hours.

Modern repertories can be obtained for computers. This convenience leaves more time for the most important part of the process, taking a good case and finding the right rubrics to put into the computer program. Now, the once tedious, time-consuming job of cross-referencing the remedies takes only moments.

### Cross-Referencing

When we *cross-reference* remedies in the various rubrics we have chosen, we are looking for remedies that are common to as many rubrics as possible. For instance, if we have chosen 5 rubrics, we would first like to see any remedies that are common to all 5 rubrics, next those that are found in 4 of 5 etc. That is the process of *repertorization* and it is used to yield a list of promising remedies that we can then look up in our Materia Medicas. I will explain that step in a later section.

### Choosing Rubrics

It is important to remember that the outcome of a repertorization is only as good as the rubrics you choose to use. Remember, the computer is only a tool. The old adage "garbage in, garbage out" applies here.

In *paragraph 14* of the *Organon*, Hahnemann says, *"There is nothing morbid that is curable which does not make itself known by means of marked signs and symptoms."* Yet, all signs and symptoms are not created equal. I talk about taking cases in a later chapter, but remember that symptoms are changes in the mind or body that cause discomfort to the organism. That discomfort is manifested distinctly in each individual person, and indicates a change in the vital force. A symptom indicates disharmony or dis-ease of the whole organism.

Symptoms are produced in the body, by the vital force in the process of curing the organism. Symptoms manifest themselves in a pattern, and the production of symptoms and the recognition of this pattern show us what remedy is required to cure the organism by returning the vital force to balance. The repertory helps us to represent these symptoms and therefore find a list of potentially curative remedies. Choosing the right rubrics to describe a well-taken case is probably the hardest thing to do in Homeopathy.

# Chapter V

## Symptoms in Homeopathy

### The Patient's Story

When Homeopaths take a case, we let the patient tell their story. Nurses understand the value of a good history given in the words of the patient. When assessing a patient, Nurses can sift through the information given and make an evaluation about what is relevant in that patient's history. Likewise, it is the job of the Homeopath to take an excellent case and then to decide what is unique to each presentation. Case taking is the Homeopath's attempt to elicit not only a detailed story of the course of the patient's illness, but also to achieve a complete understanding of the whole patient. This detailed questioning leads to the choice of symptoms obtained from the patient's story that will be repertorized and represent the case as a whole.

Symptoms describe the individuality and susceptibility of the patient. The symptom picture that we see in our case taking is particular to an individual and to how their vital force is reacting to the disease. In Homeopathy, there are different types of symptoms. Some symptom categories are more important than others. Homeopaths organize symptoms in specific ways and give them hierarchical importance, as follows.

---

**Hierarchy of Symptoms**

| Importance ↑ |
|---|
| Strange, rare and peculiar symptoms |
| Mental-emotional symptoms |
| General symptoms |
| Particular symptoms |
| Common symptoms |

Table 5:1

---

Although there are many similarities between the Nursing assessment and Homeopathic case taking, there are some significant differences as well. Nurses are involved with getting the medical and social history of the patient, which is generally taken at face value. Good physical examination should be part of the Homeopathic intake as it is in the Nursing evaluation. The use made of the symptoms reported is quite different for the two disciplines. A symptom that may be highly significant to a Homeopath may not be useful at all for a Nurse. Let me elaborate on this by discussing the different types of symptoms in Homeopathy.

**Patient Symptoms**

The following lists and defines the different type of symptoms that a patient can have. There are four ways to classify symptoms. To avoid confusion please remember that categories of symptoms were developed for teaching purposes. Some symptoms that you find in patients may fit in two categories at the same time. A person may have what would be considered a **prescribing symptom** that is at the same time **strange, rare and peculiar.**

The *first group* includes,

**Presenting symptoms:** This is the chief complaint of the patient. These include *prescribing* and *concomitant symptoms* discussed below. Presenting symptoms are very important because the patient is telling you what is wrong and why they have come in. The patient is also giving you a description of how these symptoms progressed and what is important around them.

**Prescribing symptoms:** These symptoms make us take notice because they are unusual. You would expect a person who sweats a lot to get thirsty, but if a person is sweating all the time and is never thirsty that is unusual and can lead to the correct remedy. So, prescribing symptoms have some manifestation in the patient that is not quite expected or on track with the physical symptoms that they are manifesting.

**Concomitant symptoms:** These are symptoms that are associated with or are seen in conjunction with other symptoms. They would be generally *unrelated* to the original symptom i.e. "Whenever I get a headache my feet sweat." Concomitant symptoms are symptoms that you would not necessarily associate with the symptom that it is accompanying. Again, for instance, fever is generally accompanied by sweat. But fever is not generally accompanied by diarrhea. You would expect urinary frequency to accompany symptoms of pain in the bladder, but you would not necessarily expect urinary frequency every time someone had a sinus infection. In these instances, diarrhea and urinary frequency would be considered concomitant symptoms.

The *second group* includes,
**Subjective symptoms:** Very much like Nursing, these are statements that the patient makes about their condition i.e. "I am always tired." Subjective symptoms (and *objective symptoms*) are important in that they allow you to find out how the patient feels about their condition, which, in turn, is important for the prescription of the remedy.

**Objective symptoms:** Again, like in Nursing, these are things that the practitioner notes i.e. blood pressure, or bruising. Objective symptoms are scientific symptoms that you can verify by observation.

The *third group* includes,
**Characteristic symptoms:** These may apply to either the patient or the remedy: "Every time I get sick in any way, I get a nose bleed." A characteristic symptom is a pattern of illness that we see expressed by the vital force and may precede any illness for that particular patient. Characteristic symptoms describe a constellation of symptoms used by Homeopaths to describe a pattern that may be seen in either the patient, the remedy, or both. This is the pattern that must be matched in order to find the correct remedy that will cure the case. For example, a person may get a headache and slight dizziness before a cold or gastrointestinal flu or a bladder infection. The headache and

dizziness are the characteristic symptom of that patient and will be reflected in the remedy that that patient receives.

The *fourth group* is:
**Strange, rare, and peculiar symptoms (SRPs):** These, like *characteristic symptoms* can refer either to the patient or to the remedy. SRPs are symptoms that you would not commonly find and would not expect to have happen in the normal course of events. SRPs can arise on any of the planes: physical, mental, or emotional. Symptoms like "laughs at serious things," or "faintness after urination" would be considered SRPs. Case taking is the art of filtering through symptoms to find what is most significant and specific to the patient, and what will most likely lead to the correct remedy choice and cure. Thus, SRPs are very important because they are the very finest of fine-tuning that leads you to a remedy when you see this picture in a patient.

The patient, of course, states the symptom to the Homeopath but there can also be some remedies that may contain the offered symptom. For example, if a patient came to you with a bladder infection and complained of all the usual symptoms and then told you his urine smelled like violets, then that would be unusual in the context of a bladder infection. That would be strange/rare/peculiar for the patient. There is a remedy *Terebinthina*, which in the repertory has under the **Urinary** section, *odor of violets*. It would be a good idea to look at that remedy closely when making a choice.

Within these four categories of symptoms we have in each:

**General symptoms**, which refer to the body as a whole, or to a metabolic process such as respiration. General symptoms usually can be repertorized in the section of the repertory called "Generalities." They refer to a general problem with the organism. For instance, "I get short of breath with exertion," "I sweat in my sleep at night," or "I'm hungry when I wake up in the morning." General symptoms are usually subjective in nature.

**Mental symptoms**, which are those that deal with the thought processes. Memory and concentration or problems with perception are included here.

**Emotional symptoms** are those symptoms that describe how a patient feels: "I'm sad all the time."

Mental and emotional symptoms encompass any symptoms that arise from temperament. They include dreams, delusions, disturbances in understanding or will, concentration, or any emotional symptoms at all.

**Particular symptoms** are symptoms that refer to a specific part of the body: "My hands are always cold," or "I have palpitations every time I sneeze." Sometimes particular symptoms are very important if they are raised to the level of an SRP but, generally, they do not tell us about the whole organism, so they are not as important as some of the other symptoms.

**Common symptoms** are those symptoms that are commonly associated with diseases: "I have a cold and I'm sneezing and my nose runs constantly." These represent the most common or universal expressions of an illness and thus are the least specific and least helpful in our quest to finding a remedy.

I realize that the variety of symptom classification and symptom hierarchy in Homeopathy can get a little confusing. Remember, that for the Homeopath, symptoms are the lifeblood of a case. Small nuances are important. Homeopaths see, for instance, each asthma attack as a separate entity. To us each person has his or her special way of presenting his or her asthma attack. Finding out what is special about each presentation leads us to the proper medication. Whereas for Nurses time is an important factor when taking a history, Homeopaths must take their time when taking the case. Homeopaths cannot stop talking to a patient until we get all the facts we need to repertorize the case. I know that this is hard to believe in this day of 7-minute patient visits, but there you have it.

Finally, to reiterate, within the various categories of the hierarchy of symptoms one may find symptoms that have more than one attribute. For example, a symptom may be concomitant *and* strange, rare and peculiar. Once again, I understand that this may seem very confusing at first, but it is how Homeopathy is done, and probably why many do not do it. When a person takes the time to learn to do Homeopathy properly, it is extremely rewarding both for the practitioner and the patient.

# Chapter VI

## Materia Medica

**Remedy Pictures**

The term *Materia Medica* refers both to the body of remedies used in homeopathic practice, and the books that describe these medications. When I use the term Materia Medica without the "s," I am referring to the whole of the homeopathic pharmacopia. Materia Medicas, with the "s," are books that contain the different remedy pictures. The remedy picture is a detailed rendition of both the findings of proving and the clinical observation of homeopaths in practice. Further on in this chapter we will talk about how these pictures are presented in various Materia Medica. Usually, the remedies are compiled in alphabetical order and include both a description of the remedy and all the symptoms that are associated with them, in an order reminiscent of the organization of the repertory.

Important, well-studied remedies are called **polycrests**. There are about one hundred of these remedies. The polycrests remedies represent the most common reaction of the vital force to many conditions. For instance, most people who drink too much alcohol tend to have a hangover. Hangovers in most people include headache, nausea, and sensitivity to light, to touch, to smells, irritability, possibly some nausea and vomiting. This is a very common pattern and we see it reflected in a remedy called *Nux Vomica*. When we see those symptoms in a patient and we give Nux Vomica, it will clear the hangover.

Not all people, of course, present with a hangover in the same way. Some people with a hangover may be achy, very short tempered, and much, much worse if they move. These people are presenting with a different picture than the *Nux Vomica*, one that is more like *Bryonia*. So, if you gave them the *Nux Vomica* just because they had a hangover, it would not work. But, when you took the case and found that the remedy was *Bryonia,* the remedy would work perfectly well.

Polycrests are generally representative of whole organisms. They may have tissue affinities, for instance, *Lycopodium* has an affinity for the gastrointestinal tract, while *Ignatia* has sensitivity for the nervous system. But, in general, the polycrests can be represented through the whole body. Other, less well-studied remedies are referred to as *smaller remedies*. They tend to have a more limited range of action and generally have specific tissue affinities. For instance, *Equisetum* has an affinity for the urinary tract.
Another category of remedies is **nosodes**. Nosodes are remedies potentized from the products of disease. *Tuberculinum*, for instance is potentized from the Tubercular bacillus. Although not well represented in our repertories, these very important remedies are critical to homeopathic practice. They are the foundational remedies that represent miasmatic states. In fact they are so powerful that they are considered prescription medications and cannot be used by a practitioner without prescriptive authority.

### Common Materia Medicas

Like repertories, there are a number of Material Medicas. Not all Materia Medica contain all remedies. Most Materia Medicas do have all the polycrests, and some Materia Medicas contain small remedies that have not been proven. Modern Materia Medicas contain remedies that are being proven now, like chocolate and neon, and some of the other noble gasses.

Until about ten years ago, the two most common Materia Medica in general use were *Lectures and Homeopathic Materia Medica* by J.T. Kent, my personal favorite, and *Homeopathic Materia Medica* by W. Boerke. Once again, these were written a long time ago and the language is a little bit archaic, and some of the terms may be unfamiliar to people not conversant with old-time terms in medicine. Over the last ten years, maybe fifteen, Materia Medicas have been expanded to include new provings and new remedies.

Some of the most popular Materia Medicas now days are: *Portraits in Homeopathic Medicines* by Katherine R. Colter, in two volumes, *Desktop Guide* by Roger Morrison, *Homeopathic Remedy Guide* by Robin Murphy, *Homeopathy and the Elements* by Yan Shelton, and many more. These do not replace the old standards by Boerke, Clark and Kent, but they expand on the knowledge that these old Homeopaths gave us.

There are some Materia Medicas that are organized by physical pathologies such as *The Desktop Companion,* by Roger Morrison, and *The Homeopathic Emergency Guide.* There is a temptation to use these as a regular medical or pharmaceutical text for prescribing in a "this for that" fashion. However, you will find that there are good descriptions of the pictures of remedies used in certain disease entities that will be very helpful to the practiced prescriber.

In the Materia Medicas we will not always see every repertory section represented with symptoms from the provings. As we discussed earlier, small remedies such as *Equisetum* have affinities for one or two organ systems. So we would expect to find a short description of the remedy and maybe only symptoms under one or two headings, Mind, Bladder and Kidney. No symptoms have been reported in the proving or found in clinical practice that involves any other part of the organism for this remedy.

## Materia Medica: Sample Entry

Here is the Materia Medica for the remedy *Cinchona officinalis* from W. Boericke *Homeopathic Materia Medica and Repertory.*

**CINCIAONA OFFICINALIS**

**(Peruvian Bark - China)**

*Debility* from exhausting discharges, from loss of vital fluids, together with a nervous *erethism*, calls for this remedy. Periodicity is most marked. Sensitive to draughts. Seldom indicated in the earlier stages of acute disease. Chronic gout. Chronic suppurative pyelitis. Postoperative gas pains, no relief from passing it.

**Mind**.-Apathetic, indifferent, disobedient, taciturn, despondent. Ideas crowd in mind; prevent sleep. Disposition to hurt other people's feelings. Sudden crying and tossing about.

**Head**.-As if skull would burst. Sensation as if brain were balancing to and fro, and striking against skull, receiving great pain. [*Sulph.*; *Sulph. ac.*] Intense *throbbing* of head and carotids. Spasmodic headache in vertex, with subsequent pain, as if bruised in sides of head. Face flushed after hæmorrhages, or sexual excesses, or loss of vital fluids. Relieved from pres- sure and warm room. Scalp sensitive; worse combing hair. Aches worse in open air, from temple to temple. Worse by contact, current of air, stepping. Dizzy when walking.

**Eyes**.-Blue color around eyes. Hollow eyes. Yellowish selerotica. Black specks, bright dazzling illusions; night blindness in anæmic retina. Spots before eyes. Photophobia. Distortion of eyeballs. Intermittent ciliary neuralgia. *Pressure in eyes*. Amaurosis; scalding lachrymation.

**Ears**.-*Ringing* in ears. External ear sensitive to touch. Hearing sensitive to noise. Lobules red and swollen.

**Nose**.-Checked catarrh. Easily bleeding from nose, especially on rising. Coryza, sneezing, watery discharge. Violent dry sneezing. Cold sweat about nose.

**Face**.-Sallow complexion. Face bloated; red.

**Mouth**.-Toothache; better pressing teeth firmly together, and by warmth. Tongue coated thick, dirty; tip burns, succeeded by ptyalism. Bitter taste. Food tastes too salty.

**Stomach**.-Tender, cold. Vomiting of undigested food. Slow digestion. Weight after eating. Ill effects of tea. Hungry without appetite. Flat taste. Darting pain crosswise in hypogastric region. Milk disagrees. Hungry longing for food, which lies undigested. *Flatulence; belching* of bitter fluid or regurgitation of food *gives no relief*; worse eating fruit. *Hiccough*. Bloatedness better by movement.

**Abdomen**.-Much flatulent colic; better bending double. *Tympanitic abdomen*. Pain in right hypochondrium. *Gallstone colic*. [Triumfetta semitriloba.] Liver and spleen swollen and enlarged. Jaundice. Internal coldness of stomach and abdomen. Gastroduodenal catarrh.

**Stool**.-Undigested, frothy, yellow; painless; worse at night, after meals, during hot weather, from *fruit*, milk, beer. Very weakening, with much flatulence. Difficult even when soft.[ *Alum.; Plat.*]

**Male.**-Excited lascivious fancy. Frequent emissions, followed by great weakness. Orchitis.

**Female.--**Menses too early. *Dark clots and abdominal distention*. Profuse menses with pain. Desire too strong. Bloody leucorrhœa. Seems to take the place of the usual menstrual discharge. Painful heaviness in pelvis.

**Respiratory**. - Influenza, with debility. Cannot breathe with head low. Labored, slow respiration; constant choking. *Suffocative catarrh; rattling in chest*; violent, hacking cough *after every meal*. Hæmorrhage from lungs. Dyspnœa, sharp pain in left lung. Asthma; worse damp weather.

**Heart.**-Irregular with weak rapid beats followed by strong, hard beats. Suffocative attacks, syncope; anæmia and dropsy.

**Back.**-Sharp pains across kidneys, worse movement and at night. Knife-like pains around back. (D. MacFarlan.)

**Extremities.**-*Pains in limbs and joints*, as if sprained; *worse, slight touch*; hard pressure relieves. Sensation as of a string around limb. Joints swollen; very sensitive, with dread or open air. Great debility, trembling, with numb sensation. Averse to exercise; sensitive to touch. Weariness of joints; worse, mornings and when sitting.

**Skin**.-*Extreme sensitiveness to touch*, but hard pressure *relieves*. *Coldness*; much sweat. One hand ice cold, the other warm. Anasarea. [*Ars.; Apis*.] *Dermatitis*; erysipelas. Indurated glands, scrofulous ulcers and caries.

**Sleep**.-Drowsiness. Unrefreshing or constant stupor. Wakens early. Protracted sleeplessness. Anxious, frightful dreams with confused consciousness on waking, so that the dream cannot be rid of and fear of dream remains. Snoring, especially with children.

**Fever**.-Intermittent, paroxysms anticipate; return every week. All stages well marked. Chill generally in forenoon, commencing in breast; thirst before chill, and little and often. Debilitating night-sweats. Free perspiration caused by every little exertion, especially on single parts. Hay fever, watery coryza, pain in temples.

**Modalities**.-*Worse, slightest touch*. Draught of air; every other day; loss of vital fluids; at night; *after eating;* bending over. *Better*, bending double; hard pressure; open air; warmth.

**Relationship**.-Antidotes: *Arn.; Ars.; Nux; Ipec.*

Compare: *Quinidin*-(Paroxysmal tachycardia and *auricular fibrillation*. Heart is slowed, and the auriculo-ventricular conduction time is lengthened. Dose 1/2 grain t.i.d.) *Cephalanthus* -Button Bush- Intermittent fever, sore throat, rheumatic symptoms, vivid dreams) - *Ars.; Cedron; Nat. sulph. Cydonia vulgaris* -Quince (supposed to be of use to strengthen the sexual organs and stomach).

Complementary: *Ferrum; Calc. phos.*

**Dose.-**Tincture, to thirtieth potency.

You will notice how complete the picture of this remedy is. Indeed this is the first remedy Hahnemann proved. It has been used as a homeopathic medication from the beginning. Note how detailed and specific it is. We know a lot about this remedy and have a lot of clinical experience with it. Once you see it in clinical practice you will never forget it.

## Matching Patient Pattern to Remedy

I would like to clarify here, once again, that Homeopathy is not a "this for that" kind of prescription medicine. There are not remedies that are "for" bladder infections. There are not remedies that are "for" headaches. There are remedies that may be more prone to have head symptoms in them, or gastrointestinal symptoms in them, for instance, but it is most important to *match the pattern of the patient to the pattern in the remedy*. This is why Homeopathy fails for a lot of practitioners, specifically, those accustomed to a list of medications that are "for" certain diagnoses. Homeopathy just does not work that way; you must take the case and match the symptoms to the remedy in order to be successful.

The Materia Medicas are used in conjunction with the repertory to find the similimum in the case. Good repertorization leaves you with a choice of the remedies to read and the remedy that comes up first in your repertorization is not always the remedy that is going to cure the case. Because we cannot know everything when we take a case, because we cannot make rubrics that exactly explain the situation, because we cannot repertorize perfectly, we cannot necessarily take the first remedy that comes up. What we have to do is read the first ten or fifteen remedies that come up with repertorization and find the remedy that most closely fits the case on the mental, emotional and physical planes. Let me sum up the process.

---

**Using Materia Medica**

- Take the case.
- Organize the case: What are the important themes and symptoms of the case?
- Find the Rubrics that best describe the themes and symptoms of the case.
- Repertorize the case.
- Read the first ten remedies and find a match.

Table 6:1

---

The practice of Homeopathy can certainly can be frustrating and time consuming, that is part of the reason that many people do not choose to pursue it. But if the right remedy is found, it will start the patient in the direction of cure every time! To be a successful Homeopath, the practitioner must be very, very familiar with Materia Medica, and with the keynotes involved in the patterns of the remedy, together with the use of the repertory. Now that we understand the tools of Homeopathy, it is time to talk about how to take a case.

# Chapter VII

## Case Taking

### Patient Focus

The patient is the focus of the Homeopathic process; without the patient, Homeopathy is pretty much a meaningless pursuit. We have already looked at both major tools used by Homeopaths, the Repertory and Materia Medicas. We have also talked a little about symptoms and their relevance to the case taking process. Case taking is probably the part of Homeopathy that nurses can relate to best. Nursing histories are an important part of patient care because they include both the present complaints of the case and the events leading to it -not merely the physical symptoms presented. A thorough nursing history gives other practitioners a better understanding of the patient that hopefully translates into better care.

In much the same way, Homeopaths, through case taking, strive to get a complete picture of the patient. They ask specific question in their uniquely Homeopathic way in order to round out the picture, which will eventually allow them to accurately prescribe a medicine that will cure the case.

### Acute Cases and Constitutional Cases

In Homeopathy as an Allopathic medicine, there are two different criteria for cases, the acute case and the chronic case or *constitutional case* as it is referred to.

The acute case in Homeopathy is one that reflects the state of the patient *at that moment in time*, physically, mentally and emotionally. Whether it is the result of an injury or some acute illness, acute cases represent the state of the vital force as it responds to any disruption that it finds itself dealing with. This acute response may or may not have anything to do with the person's usual constitutional state.

For good homeopathic prescribing, though, it is important to note that each individual's response to an environmental stressor is appropriate to his constitutional state so that when somebody gets a cold, depending upon their constitutional type, they will display different symptoms of that cold in an acute situation. This really has to be taken into consideration when we are looking for a remedy in a case.

A *constitutional case* –or chronic case, on the other hand, is usually the result of a long illness or condition that is part of the patient's entire picture. It involves not only a physical complaint, if any, but also a mental evaluation and an emotional plane evaluation. It is important for the Homeopath to look at the entire patient in order to fit a remedy that is going to cover the whole picture. Later, when we talk about case analysis we will look at a few cases and the difference will become very clear.

A word of caution is due here. As with Nursing, it is important for the practitioner taking the history to be an unbiased observer and ask questions in such a way that the patient will not be lead to the answer that *we* would like to have. This is always tricky ground for new homeopathic practitioners. Usually their knowledge of Materia Medica is not broad and it is limited mostly to polycrests. Thus, novice homeopathic practitioners may ask questions from their patients and start to get a preconceived notion of what remedy they think is going to be appropriate. So, they ask question that will direct a patient to that remedy. This leads to many false prescriptions in homeopathic practices. It is the job of the Homeopath, indeed, as it is the job of the Nurse, to take an unbiased, thorough history.

## Observation

In the effort for good, unbiased, and through case taking, observation is one of the most critical aspects and something that may be sacrificed in the rush to treat as many patients as possible in a limited amount of time. Often, observation tells us as much, if not more than laboratory tests, or even a physical exam. How does the patient walk in? How do they sit? Are they in pain when they move? Do they interact with you in a straightforward way? Will they look us in the eyes when they answer a question? The basic skill of observation is as important in Homeopathy as it is in Nursing.

Homeopathically speaking, we can learn a tremendous amount about the patient by observing; even by noting subtleties such as the type and color of clothing that they choose to wear. Observation gives us details that sometimes the patient will forget to tell us. These subtleties have been part of their life for so long that they forget that they exist. Hahnemann explains this very well in the *Organon*, in *aphorism 95*:

> *"Chronically ill patients become so accustomed to their long suffering that they pay little or not attention to the smaller, often very characteristic accompanying bafflements which are so decisive in singling out the remedy. They view them as almost part of their natural state, nearly mistaking them for health, whose true feeling they have fairly well forgotten during the course of their fifteen to twenty year long suffering. It hardly occurs to them to believe that these accompanying symptoms, these remaining smaller or greater deviations from the healthy state, could have a connection with their main malady."*

**Getting Started**

For homeopathic practice, the setting of the interview is also very important. Remember that these patients may be sitting in your office for an hour to an hour and a half, sometimes two hours. So, it is important that the setting be comfortable, quiet and non-threatening.

Once started, there are multiple ways to proceed. Practitioners have their own way of taking a case. Some practitioners sit and simply let the patient talk. They take down every word the patient says. This method is quite time consuming and leaves you with reams and reams of paper.

However, it gives you tremendous insight into the workings of the patient's mind. If your style is to ask questions, then it is probably always better to ask the open-ended questions. Instead of saying, "Do you have constipation? Yes or No." It is better to say, "Do you have any problems with your bowels?" This way the patient can tell you the story in his own words and you can clarify small details later, if you need to.

### Chief Complaint and Modalities

I usually start my case-taking by asking the patient, "What brought you in today?" This would correspond with the chief complaint in allopathic case taking. Once the patient has said what they have to say about their chief complaint, it is important to get the **modalities.** Modalities are the conditions that modify a symptom. They include things like the location of the problem, what makes it better, what makes it worse, how often it occurs. They round out the picture of the chief complaint and give us something to go by when we choose the rubrics that will describe our case for repertorization. A similar tool in Nursing would be the mnemonic *PQRST*: Provoking/Palliative, Quality/Quantity, Radiation/Region, Severity/associated Symptoms, and Timing/Temporal sequence.

### Causation

Causation, or ideology is the next very important part of the case taking. The chief complaint had to start at some time and it had to happen for a reason. Sometimes the patient does not know this reason, or they will say something like, "Oh, well this happened, but my doctor said that wasn't important at the time." Always ask questions about that event. Ideology is extremely important in Homeopathy and the phrase, "never well since" can lead us to a remedy that fits the case perfectly.

**Review of Systems**

As in Nursing, it is important to do a review of systems, even if the chief complaint does not involve any other organ system than the one talked about by the patient. The way the person functions generally in their body is extremely important to the choice of remedy. You may uncover other problems that they simply do not consider problems, but will be confirmatory when it comes to finding the correct remedy in the Materia Medica.

A review of systems includes questions about the different planes (see Figure 3:1). Mental symptoms are the symptoms that describe how the patient thinks and concentrates. It is important to know the way the person thinks and the kinds of things they remember. Are they linear thinkers? Are they logical? Are they more left brained, more right brained? How do they approach the world in their mental plane? Do they sometimes feel fuzzy in thought? Is their concentration affected? Do they have a hard time sticking to task? All these things are extremely important to know about the mental plane and the thought process of a person. If a person is more seriously ill and has some kind of a mental plane diagnosis, it is important to know whether they hear voices, whether they hallucinate. These are all mental plane, not emotional plane problems, and are indicative of deep-seated illnesses.

Emotional plane pictures can be some of hardest, or, in some cases, the easiest pictures to get. Open-ended questions like, "Tell me about yourself." will illicit information that the patient probably has not been able to say to people in a very long time. As healthcare consumers, we are not used to having a doctor ask us how we feel, and that in itself is therapeutic for many patients. They come into our office, they sit down, and they unload a tremendous amount of pent-up energy. Just the opportunity to get those things off their chest makes them feel a whole lot better. These are of course, bedside secrets that Nurses have been practicing for years. Sometimes I think that about 70% of the therapeutic effect of Homeopathy is just allowing the patient to tell their story. Finding the Similimum, the right remedy, will make the patient feel 100% better. We need to know not just how they feel, but why they feel the way they feel. Not just what they do, but why they do it, because the crux of case taking for repertorization is in finding the why and wherefore of the symptoms that the patient's talked to us about. Like the famous detectives, we want to know what, where, when, why and how.

There will be questions that overlap the boundaries of the physical plane, mental and emotional planes. These include the areas of sexuality, and sleep. Once we start looking at patients homeopathically, it becomes very obvious that the physical plane, the mental plane and the emotional plane interact with each other all the time.

In the allopathic system it is easy to separate things into categories, but the problem with chronic disease, is that its etiology may not be reflected in the chief complaint. In fact, it very often resides somewhere other than the symptom picture suggests. For instance, if a person comes in complaining of insomnia, and we just give them a sleeping pill and never ask when it started or what was happening at the time it started, and we find out later that the person has recently experienced the death of her mother, the failure of her marriage, and her children leaving home all at the same time, it would then not surprise us that sleep is a problem. Just giving a sleep medication is not going to take care of that problem in the long run. We see similar situations when dealing with sexual dysfunction.

A man may come in complaining of impotence, but has been on beta-blockers for a long period of time. Over the last six months he has been unable to have an erection. He states he loves his wife of 25 years, and that their sex life was great before the medication. It is fairly obvious that the problem is on the physical plane and the medication is the culprit. However, the person may need the medication and cannot get off of it, and so some other solution to the problem will have to happen. On the other hand, a woman many come in complaining of lack of sexual desire, and you question her further and find out that her husband has been cheating on her and that every since she found that out she just has had no desire to sleep with him. In this instance, the problem would not be on the physical plane. The above examples illustrate the same chief complain with different etiologies discovered by a thorough review of systems.

**History and Lifestyle**

Similar to Nursing, in the course of case taking we also want to know past medical history, family history and any medications that the person is taking. In addition we will also ask about patient lifestyle. Asking about lifestyle is important because it tells us about the concept of "obstacles to cure." In *Aphorism 94*, Hahnemann tells us,

> *"While inquiring into the state of chronic disease, carefully ponder and scrutinize the particular affairs of the patient to find out what there is in them that may arouse or maintain disease and whose removal may further recovery."*

These are words to live by. For many years in allopathic medicine, patients with lung disease who smoked were not cautioned to stop smoking. If you have emphysema, smoking cigarettes is a serious impediment to cure and the Homeopath really cannot do a whole lot for a patient that is smoking while they are being treated for something like emphysema. Again, like Nursing, inquiring about lifestyle will help us to educate our patients about what they can do to participate in their own wellness and health maintenance after we have analyzed our case and decided which remedy to give.

**Homeopathic Considerations**

Other questions or more homeopathic considerations include perspiration (Does the person perspire easily? Do they perspire too much? ), temperature (Are they hot? Are they cold?), food and water (Do they have thirst? Are they thirst less? What source of foods do they like? What foods do they dislike?). These considerations are less common in Nursing practice yet in Homeopathy they play a part in finding the remedy. Remember that the key to the correct remedy may be found in a symptom or modality that is as we say, strange, rare or peculiar. These are the kinds of questions that may lead us to these insights.

## Organizing The Case

Case taking generates a lot of information, thus, efficient organization of the data can be problematic. In order to succeed, there has to be a way to highlight the various parts of the case that you think are important. Traditionally, Homeopaths have underlined the parts of the case that they feel are most pertinent to the whole picture presented by the patient. One underline is something to look at, two underlines is something that the patient stated, and three underlines is something they stated emphatically.

I like to take a case using headings on the margin, with information about those headings beside them in the body of the text. Then I can underline or highlight the sections that seem important to me at the time. That way, when I go back to organize the case, I do not have to re-read it through multiple times in order to get the information as organized as I would like it to be. The object of organizing a case and assessing a case is to get it into a concise and manageable form from which rubrics can be generated.

In *Chapter V,* we talked about symptoms and the importance of each type of symptom in case taking. What we do next is to organize our case into three categories or "boxes" corresponding each to the Physical Plane, Mental Plane and Emotional Plane. We classify each symptom that is important to our case into these three categories. We organize our case considering each plane of the patient and prioritize the information in each section using the hierarchy of symptoms we have noted in previous chapters.

For example, in the Physical Plane we may have only presenting symptoms, we have the chief complaint. Some of the symptoms may have concomitant symptoms, some of those symptoms may be subjective, and some of them may turn out to be characteristic symptoms. We would go about organizing this by placing those symptoms down in the "physical plane box."

If the patient has mental plane symptoms they will manifest themselves as loss of memory or poor concentration. A patient may complain of "fuzzy thinking." He may forget words. Any complaint that involves the thought process is organized under "mental plane box." This includes such serious symptoms as hearing voices. Schizophrenia is a mental disease, although it can affect the emotional plane. If a person has no problem in the mental plane, if they can think and concentrate without problems, then there is not going to be anything in that category or box.

We do the same in the Emotional Plane, but in this plane we try to not only elicit the feelings of the patient but also the motivation for the reaction. We think of these in terms of "concepts," because concepts have to do with rationales for actions. So, perhaps the person overall is sad, or perhaps the person overall is angry, and from anger comes the symptoms that the patient elicits. These emotional concepts are reflected in remedy pictures. Some remedies reflect specific motivation and the actions of a patient come from these basic motivations.

For example, the actions of a patient needing *Arsenicum album* are motivated by fear that she will never have enough of anything. This fear makes her want to control her world. Everything she does stems from that concept. So, for instance when you see fastidiousness in a patient you have to ask why is this happening? Is she protective of her goods, like *Arsenicum* or is she afraid of what others will think of her like *Natrum Muriaticum*? This can be the trickiest part of case taking, especially for the novice. The following cases should serve to illustrate this point.

# Chapter VIII

## Case Studies

### Illustrating the Case

The following three cases should help clarify the case taking process. The first two cases would be considered acute cases. They are both viral labrynthitis. The third case, though, has an acute presentation, but is actually a chronic recurrent cystitis and needs to be treated in a constitutional way.

### Case One

A thirty-five year old female comes in complaining of vertigo for three weeks. Onset occurred after a bout of influenza. She had seen her allopathic physician and was given antibiotics with the flu symptoms, and when vertigo appeared, she got an antihistamine. Neither of these treatments has helped the vertigo. She has a headache, mostly in her temples and she says that she "can't think straight." She has ringing in her ears and when she stands she feels dizzy and has to balance to the left side. She has no other symptoms and is a little bit anxious that this will never go away. Nothing like this has ever happened to her before.

This case is fairly simple to organize. We concentrate mostly on the vertigo symptoms, since that is the chief complaint and there does not seem to be anything else going on in the case now. So, what is pertinent is how her vertigo presents. She has a tendency to fall to the left, she has ringing in her hears, she has a headache, but this is a very common symptom and there is nothing specific that we can put into the repertorization that will really give us any help. The format below is the computer version of what had to be done by hand before the "electronic age." I think it is obvious how time consuming this process can be. This first case is very short and only two rubrics have been chosen.

When you look at the cases that follow it, you will have a greater appreciation of the work that would be involved without the computer. We will talk more about this at the end of the chapter, and the resource section will tell you how to find more information on this subject.

The rubrics I chose in this case are vertigo, fall, tendency to the left, and head, hearing, noises in ears, ringing.

### Case 1

* 1. V; Vertigo; FALL, tendency to; left, to (27)
* 2. H; Hearing; NOISES, in ears,: ringing (184)

| | | **Calc.** | **Sal-ac.** | **Nat-m.** | **Caust.** | **Bell.** | **Bor.** | **Aur.** | **Sulph.** | **Euph.** | **Stram.** | **Nat-c.** | **Nux-m.** | **Iris-foe.** | **Spig.** |
|---|---|---|---|---|---|---|---|---|---|---|---|---|---|---|---|
| **Total** | | 5 | 2 | 5 | 5 | 5 | 4 | 4 | 5 | 3 | 2 | 2 | 3 | 2 | 3 |
| **Rubrics** | | 2 | 2 | 2 | 2 | 2 | 2 | 2 | 2 | 2 | 2 | 2 | 2 | 2 | 2 |
| **Family** | | | | | | | | | | | | | | | |
| **Vertigo; FALL, tendency** | (27) | 2 | 1 | **3** | 2 | 2 | 2 | 2 | 2 | 1 | 1 | 1 | 1 | 2 | 1 |
| **Hearing; NOISES, in** | (184) | **3** | 1 | 2 | **3** | **3** | 2 | 2 | **3** | 2 | 1 | 1 | 2 | | 2 |

Table 8:1

Before we start to analyze this case let me explain what you are seeing when you look at the figure above. This repertorization was done with *MacRepertory,* a popular Homeopathy computer program (see the following section for a discussion on computer programs). The rubrics used are listed above the graph. They are numbered in the order that they were put in the program. The graph is organized as follows:

*Top Line:* Remedies that the repertorization produced.
*Total:* The numerical value derived from the addition of the numbers next to the rubrics below it.
*Rubrics:* Represents the number of rubrics in which the remedy above appeared, out of the total number chosen (in this case, *Calc* was under both rubrics chosen).
*Family:* This line is important in an analysis strategy beyond the scope of this book.
*List of rubrics used:* The lines that follow list the rubrics in the order they were put in the program. The numbers under

each remedy (1, 2 or 3) have been explained previously (see page 28). When these numbers are added vertically under each remedy they add up to the number found under *Total.*

As you can see, the repertorization has given us some remedies. The first one is *Calcaria carbonicum,* the second one is *Salicylic Acidum*, the third *Natrum Muriaticum*, and *Causticum, Belladonna, Borax, Orum*, etc. You will remember from *Chapter IV* that remedies found under rubrics are in **bold,** *italic,* or regular print. These correspond with a number value in the example above, 3 for **bold,** 2 for *italic,* 1 for regular. This way you can see not only that the remedy appeared under that rubric, but how often it was represented in the provings. In the repertorization above, you can see that *Calc. c* is the first remedy that is listed. Remember that you must now go to the Materia Medica and read about the remedies that appear in the repertorization. When you read *Calc. c* it is obvious that this is not the correct remedy. But, after you read *Salicylicum acidum*, you can see that this case is a *Salicylicum acidum* case. It has the ringing in the ears, it has vertigo falling to the left, and, interestingly enough, it also has ill effects of influenza. So, I chose this remedy. I gave the lady a 30c potency that she could take every three hours as needed until there was any change in her vertigo. It took her three doses of the remedy and the vertigo never came back. Here is the Materica Medica for *Sal-ac*

### SALICYLICUM ACIDUM
**(Salicylic Acid)**

The symptoms point to its use in rheumatism, dyspepsia, and *Meniere's disease.* Prostration after influenza; also tinnitus aurium and deafness. Hæmaturia.

**Head.**-Vertigo; tendency to fall to left side. Headache; confusion in head on rising suddenly. Incipient coryza. Piercing pain in temples.

**Eyes.**-Retinal hemorrhage. Retinitis after influenza, also albuminuric.

**Ears.**-*Roaring and ringing in ear.* Deafness, with vertigo.

**Throat.**- Sore, red and swollen. Pharyngitis; swallowing difficult.

**Stomach.**- *Canker sores*, with burning soreness and fetid breath. *Flatulence; hot, sour belching.* Putrid fermentation. *Fermentative dyspepsia.* Tongue purplish, leaden-colored, foul breath.

**Stools.**-Putrid diarrhœa; gastrointestinal derangements, especially in children; stools like green frog's spawn. [*Magn. carb.*] Pruritus ani.

**Extremities.**-Knees swollen and painful. Acute articular rheumatism; worse, touch and motion, profuse sweat. Pain shifts. Sciatica, burning pain; worse at night. Copious foot sweat and ill affects where suppressed.

**Skin**.-Itching vesicles and pustules; better by scratching. Sweat without sleep. Urticaria. Hot and burning skin. Purpura. Herpes zoster. Necrosis and softening of bones.

**Relationship**.- Compare: *Salol* (rheumatic pain in joints, with soreness and stiffness, headache over eyes; urine violet-smelling); *Colch.*; *China; Lact. ac.* Spiræa and Gaultheria contain salicyl. acid.

**Dose**.-Third

A word here about using the Materia Medica: All the symptoms that one finds in the remedy pictures seen in Materia Medica do not have to be present in all cases. Thus, even though this case did not have the skin symptoms of itching vesicles, it was still the correct remedy because its vertigo symptoms covered this case perfectly.

### Case Two

This second case is also a labrynthitis case. A forty-year old female who has had vertigo with falling for the last three weeks has been to the doctor and "they do not seem to be able to do anything about it." She says she does not really understand how it happened, "it just happened." Such events have never occurred before in her life. Our patient is really very fearful and anxious, and she is afraid she is never going to get well. She says now even little things bother her and she is always jumpy. I ask her how her vertigo started and she says the onset was quite sudden. She was walking with her sister-in-law, it was a windy, blustery, cold afternoon and from one step to another she just got dizzy. This is very unusual for her. I ask her if she has had any colds or flues. She stated that she had, in fact, had the sniffles, for a while before they had gone out for their walk. Otherwise, everything was fine. She has a tendency to fall to the right, when she falls, and she really doesn't know what to do about this. She has had antihistamines from her doctor, but they have not worked.

When you look at this case, you would think, generally that vertigo is vertigo, but once you look at the rubrics chosen for this case, you see vertigo, just general, vertigo, tendency to fall to the right, vertigo, sudden onset, and mind, fear, general, phobias, and environment, wind, general aggravates, cold aggravates. When you look at the repertorization, you see the remedies that are given are *Arsenicum, Allium cepa,*

*Lyss, Aconite, Asterium, Calcaria phosphoricum, Hepar,* and *Iris,* etc.

## Case II

1. V; Vertigo; VERTIGO, remedies (281)
* 2. V; Vertigo; VERTIGO, FALL, tendency to; right (18)
* 3. V; Vertigo; VERTIGO, SUDDEN (31)
4. M; Mind; FEAR, general, phobias (242)
5. E; Environment; WIND, general, agg.; cold, agg. (38)

| | | **Ars.** | **All-C.** | **Lyss.** | **Acon.** | **Aster.** | **Calc-p.** | **Hep.** | **Iris.** | **Caust.** | **Mill.** | **Spong.** | **Stram.** | **Rhus-t.** | **Camph.** |
|---|---|---|---|---|---|---|---|---|---|---|---|---|---|---|---|
| **Total** | | 9 | 5 | 5 | 10 | 4 | 6 | 7 | 3 | 9 | 2 | 7 | 6 | 9 | 5 |
| **Rubrics** | | 5 | 3 | 3 | 4 | 3 | 3 | 3 | 3 | 4 | 2 | 3 | 3 | 4 | 4 |
| **Family** | | | | | | | | | | | | | | | |
| **Vertigo; VERTIGO** | (281) | 2 | 1 | 1 | **3** | 2 | 2 | 2 | 1 | 2 | 1 | 2 | 2 | **3** | 2 |
| **VERTIGO, FALL, tendency** | (18) | 1 | | 1 | 2 | | | | | 2 | 1 | | | 1 | 1 |
| **V; Vertigo; SUDDEN** | (31) | 1 | | | | 1 | | | 1 | | | | 1 | | 1 |
| **Mind; FEAR, general** | (242) | **3** | 2 | 3 | **3** | 1 | **3** | 2 | 1 | 2 | | 2 | **3** | 2 | 1 |
| **Environment; WIND,** | (38) | 2 | 2 | | 2 | | 1 | **3** | | **3** | | **3** | | **3** | |

Table 8:2

When we read *Arsenicum* in the materia medicas, there is definitely the anxiety, there is also the vertigo. Even though *Arsenicum* is a three for fear, most of its fears are anxieties more than actually being afraid. And, if you know this remedy, you know it's just not right.

For *Allium cape*, you have to see a lot of runny nose, *Lyssin* is not the right remedy. *Aconitum* is the remedy of choice, and since she had had this thing for three weeks and it was looking like it was going to put a layer on her, I gave her an *Aconitum* 1M. In twenty-four hours the vertigo was gone and it has never come back. Here is the Materia Medica of *Aconitum*.

### ACONITUM NAPELLUS
### (Monkshood)

A state of fear, anxiety; anguish of mind and body. *Physical and mental restlessness*, fright, is the most characteristic manifestation of *Aconite*. *Acute, sudden, and violent invasion, with fever*, call for it. Does not want to be touched. Sudden and great sinking of strength. *Complaints and tension* caused by exposure to *dry, cold weather*, draught of cold air, checked perspiration, also complaints from *very hot weather*, especially gastro-intestinal disturbances, etc. First remedy in inflammations, inflammatory fevers. Serous membranes and muscular tissues affected markedly.

Burning in internal parts; *tingling, coldness and numbness*. Influenza. *Tension* of arteries; emotional and physical mental tension explain many, symptoms. When prescribing Aconite remember Aconite causes only functional disturbance, no evidence that it can produce tissue change -- its action is brief and *shows no periodicity*. Its sphere is in the beginning of an acute disease and not to be continued after pathological change comes. In Hyperæmia, congestion not after exudation has set in. *Influenza [Influenzin]*

**Mind.**--*Great fear, anxiety*, and worry accompany every ailment, however trivial. Delirium is characterized by unhappiness -- worry, fear, raving, rarely unconsciousness. *Forebodings and fears. Fears death* but believes that he will soon die; predicts the day. *Fears the future*, a crowd, crossing the street. *Restlessness*, tossing about. Tendency to start. Imagination acute, clairvoyance. Pains are intolerable; they drive him crazy. Music is unbearable; makes her sad. [*Ambra*.] Thinks his thoughts come from the stomach-that parts of his body are abnormally thick. Feels as if what had just been done was a dream.

**Head.**-Fullness; *heavy*, pulsating, *hot, bursting*, burning, undulating sensation. Intercranial pressure. (*Hedera Helix*.) Burning headache, as if brain were moved by boiling water [*Indigo*.]. Vertigo; *worse on rising* [*Nux. Opium*] and shaking head. Sensation on vertex as if hair were pulled or stood on end. Nocturnal furious delirium.

**Eyes**.-Red, inflamed. Feel *dry and hot*, as if sand in them. *Lids swollen, hard and red*. Aversion to light. Profuse watering after exposure to dry, cold winds, *reflection from snow, after extraction of cinders* and other foreign bodies.

**Ears**.-Very *sensitive to noises*; music is unbearable. External ear hot, red, painful, swollen. Earache. [*Cham*.] Sensation as of drop of water in left ear.

**Nose**.-*Smell acutely sensitive. Pain at root of nose*. Coryza; much sneezing; throbbing in nostrils. Hæmorrhage of bright red blood. *Mucous membrane dry, nose stopped up; dry or with but scanty watery coryza*.

**Face**.-Red, hot, flushed, swollen. One cheek red, the other pale (*Cham., Ipec.*). *On rising the red face becomes deathly pale, or he becomes dizzy. Tingling* in cheeks and numbness. Neuralgia, *especially of left side, with restlessness, tingling, and numbness*. Pain in jaws.

**Mouth**.-Numb, *dry*, and tingling. Tongue swollen; *tip tingles*. Teeth sensitive to cold. Constantly moves lower jaw as if chewing. *Gums hot and inflamed. Tongue coated white*. [*Antim. crud*.]

**Throat** --*Red, dry, constricted*, numb, prickling, burning, -Tonsils swollen and dry.

**Stomach**.-*Vomiting, with fear, heat, profuse sweat and increased urination*. Thirst for cold water. *Bitter taste* of everything except water. *Intense thirst*. Drinks, vomits, and declares he will die. Vomiting, bilious, mucous and bloody, greenish. Pressure in stomach with dyspnoæ. Hæmatemesis. Burning from stomach to esophagus.

**Abdomen**.-Hot, tense, tympanitic. *Sensitive to touch. Colic*, no position relieves. Abdominal symptoms better after warm soup. Burning in umbilical region.

**Rectum**.-Pain with nightly itching and stitching in anus. Frequent, small stool with tenesmus; *green, like chopped herbs*. White with red urine. Choleraic discharge with collapse, anxiety, and restlessness. Bleeding hæmorrhoids. [*Hamam*.] Watery diarrhœa in children. They cry and complain much, are sleepless and restless.

**Urine**.-*Scanty, red, hot, painful*. Tenesmus and. burning at neck of bladder. Burning in urethra. Urine suppressed, bloody. Anxiety always on beginning to urinate. *Retention, with screaming and restlessness*, and. handling of genitals. Renal region sensitive. Profuse urination, with profuse perspiration and diarrhoea.

**Male**.-Crawling and stinging in glans. Bruised pain in testicles, swollen, hard. Frequent erections and emissions. Painful erections.

**Female**.-Vagina dry, hot, sensitive. Menses too profuse, with nosebleed, too protracted, late. Frenzy on appearance of menses. *Suppressed from fright, cold*, in plethoric subjects. Ovaries congested and painful. Sharp shooting pains in womb. *After-pains, with fear and restlessness*.

**Respiratory**.-Constant pressure in left chest; *oppressed breathing* on least motion. *Hoarse, dry, croupy cough*; loud, labored breathing. Child grasps at throat every time he, coughs. Very sensitive to inspired air. *Shortness of breath*. Larynx sensitive. Stitches through chest. Cough, dry, short, hacking; *worse at night and after midnight*. Hot feeling in lungs. Blood comes up with hawking. Tingling in chest after cough.

**Heart**.-*Tachycardia*. Affections of the heart with pain *in left shoulder*. Stitching pain in chest. *Palpitation, with anxiety*, fainting, and *tingling* in fingers. *Pulse full, hard; tense and bounding*, sometimes intermits. Temporal and carotid arteries felt when sitting.

**Back-** Numb, stiff, painful. Crawling and tingling, as if bruised. Stiffness in nape of neck. Bruised pain between scapulæ.

**Extremilties**.- *Numbness and tingling*; shooting pains; icy coldness and insensibility of hands and feet. Arms feel lame, bruised, heavy, numb. Pain down left arm [*Cact., Crotal., Kalmia, Tobac.*] *Hot hands and cold feet*. Rheumatic inflammation of joints; worse at night; red shining swelling, very sensitive. Hip-joint and thigh feel lame, especially after lying down. Knees unsteady; disposition of foot to turn. [*Æscula*.] Weak and lax ligaments of all joints. Painless cracking of all joints. -*Bright red hypothenar eminences on both hands*. Sensation as if drops of water trickled down the thigh.

**Sleep**.-Nightmare. Nightly ravings. *Anxious dreams*. ,Sleeplessness, with restless and tossing about. [Use thirtieth potency] Starts up in sleep. Long dreams, with anxiety in chest. Insomnia of the aged.

**Skin**.-Red, hot, swollen, dry, burning. *Purpura miliaris*. Rash like measles. Gooseflesh. Formication and numbness. Chilliness and formication down back. Pruritus *relieved* by stimulants.

**Fever**.--Cold stage most marked. Cold sweat and icy coldness of face. Coldness and heat alternate. Evening chilliness soon after going to bed. *Cold waves pass through him*. *Thirst and restlessness* always present. Chilly if uncovered or touched. Dry heat, red face. Most valuable febrifuge with mental anguish, restlessness, etc. Sweat drenching, on parts lain on; relieving all symptoms.

**Modalities**.- *Better* in open air; *worse* in warm room, in evening and *night*; *worse* lying on affected side, from music, from tobacco-smoke, dry, cold winds. Vinegar in large doses is antidotal to poisonous effects.

**Relationship**.-Acids, wine and coffee, lemonade, and acid fruits modify its action. Not indicated in malarial and low fevers or hectic and pyæmic conditions, and in inflammations when they localize themselves. *Sulphur* often follows it. Compare *Cham*. and *Coffea* in *intense pain and* sleeplessness.

**Dose**.-Sixth potency for sensory affections; first to third for congestive conditions. Must be repeated frequently in acute diseases. Acon. is a rapid worker. In Neuralgias tincture of the root often preferable, one drop doses (poisonous), or again, the 30th potency according to susceptibility of the patient.

As you can see *Acon* is a well-proven and commonly used remedy. Just an interesting note, since *911*, *Aconitum* has been one of the most commonly prescribed remedies for emotional trauma suffered by patients following that event.

## Case Three

This case is a constitutional case. This twenty-seven year old female came in complaining of a bladder infection. Upon questioning, we learn that this is a recurrent problem for her. She has had bladder infections all her life. They are worse if she gets upset about something, especially if she feels that someone is disrespecting her. She is a sweet, soft-spoken young woman. She married young, at the age of seventeen to get out of an abusive home situation. She tries to please everyone so that they will like her. Apparently, her marriage has not turned out very well, as her husband is cheating on her. When she talks about it, she states that she would "just like to throw something at him" she is so angry. Review of systems is unremarkable except for a history of styes, in fact, she just got over one last week prior to the onset of the present bladder symptoms. The bladder symptoms present as a pain in the bladder and even after the bladder is empty it feels like there is still more. There is pressure in between urinations. The bladder symptoms always happen after intercourse, and there is burning pain and urinary frequency.

In this case, although the symptomology is clearly on the physical plane, the etiology of this case is in the emotional plane. Here is a person who has felt disrespected her whole life, and is terribly angry about it. She chooses to deal with her situation by being sweet and nice, trying to please everybody. This suppression of the anger that she felt she could not express lead to the physical symptoms of chronic, recurrent bladder infections and probably styes. When we repertorize this case, we have to not only take into consideration the bladder symptoms, which are important, but also the emotional plane symptoms, the mind symptoms, ailments from indignation, ailments from anger, and the other anger, anger with grief with silence and anger from indignation, and illness after anger. All of these symptoms are very important in this case.

**Case III**

*1. B; Bladder; URINATION, general; frequent, urination (187)
*2. B; Bladder; URINATION, general; painful, urination (149)
*3. B; Bladder; IRRITATION, URETHRA (12)
4. B; Bladder; CYSTITIS, inflammation, bladder; chronic (48)
5. B; Bladder; CYSTITIS, inflammation, bladder; recurrent (5)
6. M; Mind; INDIGNATION, feelings; ailments from (11)
7. E; Eyes, STYES, lower lids (12)
*8. B; Bladder, URINATION, general; incomplete, urination (29)
9. M; Mind; ANGER, general; ailments, after anger (93)
10. M; Mind; ANGER, general; grief, with silent (27)
11. M; Mind; ANGER, general; indignation, with (12)

| | | **Staph.** | **Coloc.** | **Lyc.** | **Pop.** | **Canth.** | **Nux-V.** | **Sel.** | **Puls.** | **Chim.** | **Cub.** | **Ip.** | **Plat.** |
|---|---|---|---|---|---|---|---|---|---|---|---|---|---|
| **Total** | | 26 | 15 | 18 | 4 | 10 | 14 | 7 | 13 | 7 | 4 | 7 | 8 |
| **Rubrics** | | 10 | 7 | 9 | 3 | 4 | 7 | 4 | 7 | 4 | 4 | 4 | 6 |
| **Family** | | | | | | | | | | | | | |
| **Bladder, URINATION,** | (187) | **3** | 2 | **3** | | **3** | **3** | 2 | **3** | 2 | | 2 | 1 |
| **Bladder, URINATION,** | (149) | 2 | 2 | **3** | 1 | **3** | **3** | 1 | **3** | 2 | 1 | | 1 |
| **Bladder, IRRITATION** | (12) | **3** | | | 1 | | | | | 1 | 1 | | |
| **Bladder, CYSTITIS,** | (48) | **3** | 1 | 1 | 2 | **3** | | | 2 | 2 | 1 | | |
| **Bladder, CYSTITIS,** | (5) | 1 | | 1 | | 1 | | | 1 | | | | |
| **Mind; INDIGNATION,** | (11) | **3** | 2 | 2 | | | 1 | | | | | 1 | 1 |
| **Eyes; STYES, lower lids** | (12) | | | | | | | | 1 | | | | |
| **Bladder; URINATION,** | (29) | 2 | | 2 | | | 1 | **3** | | | 1 | | |
| **Mind, ANGER, general;** | (93) | **3** | **3** | 2 | | | **3** | 1 | 2 | | | **3** | **3** |
| **Mind, ANGER, general;** | (27) | **3** | 2 | **3** | | | 1 | | 1 | | | | 1 |
| **Mind, ANGER, general;** | (12) | **3** | **3** | 1 | | | 2 | | | | | 1 | 1 |

Table 8:3

When we look at the repertorization, we see that we have *Staphysagria, Colocynthis, Lycopodium,* etc. *Staphysagria*, in this case, comes up number one and is the correct remedy. *Colocynthis* is also a remedy for ailments after anger, but it has a very different feel to it from *staphysagria*. The following are the Materia Medica for both *Staph* and *Coloc*.

## STAPHYSAGRIA
## (Stavesacre)

Nervous affections with marked irritability, diseases of the genito-urinary tract and skin, most frequently give symptoms calling for this drug. Acts on teeth and alveolar periosteum. Ill effects of anger and insults. *Sexual sins and excesses. Very sensitive.* Lacerated tissues. Pain and nervousness after extraction of teeth. Sphincters lacerated or stretched.

**Mind**.-Impetuous, *violent outbursts of passion*, hypochondriacal, sad. *Very sensitive* as to what others say about her. Dwells on sexual matters; prefers solitude. Peevish. Child cries for many things, and refuses them when offered.

**Head**.-Stupefying headache; passes off with yawning. Brain feels squeezed. Sensation of a ball of lead in forehead. Itching eruption above and behind ears. [*Oleand.*]

**Eyes**-. Heat in eyeballs, dims spectacles. *Recurrent styes. Chalazæ.* [*Platanus.*) Eyes sunken, with blue rings. Margin of lids itch. Affections of angles of eye, particularly the inner. Lacerated or incised wounds of cornea. Bursting pain in eyeballs of syphilitic iritis.

**Throat.-** *Stitches flying to the ear on swallowing, especially left.*

**Mouth**.-Toothache during menses. *Teeth black and crumbling*. Salivation, spongy gums, bleed easily. [*Merc.; Kreos.*] Submaxillary glands swollen. After eating feels sleepy. Pyorrhœa. [*Plantago.*]

**Stomach.**-Flabby and weak. Desire for stimulants. Stomach feels relaxed. *Craving for tobacco*. Canine hunger, even when stomach is full. Nausea after abdominal operations.

**Abdomen**.-Colic after anger. Hot flatus. Swollen abdomen in children, with much flatus. Colic, with pelvic tenesmus. *Severe pain following an abdominal operation*. Incarcerated flatus. Diarrhœa after drinking cold water, with tenesmus. Constipation (2 drops tincture night and morning), hæmorrhoids, with enlarged prostate.

**Male**.-Especially after self-abuse; persistent dwelling on sexual subjects. Spermatorrhœa, with sunken features; guilty look; emissions, with backache and weakness and sexual neurasthenia. Dyspnœa after coition.

**Female.**-*Parts very sensitive*, worse sitting down. [*Berb.*; *Kreos.*] *Irritable bladder in young married women*. Leucorrhœa. Prolapsus, with sinking in the abdomen; aching around the hips.

**Urinary.**--*Cystocele* (locally and internally) Cystitis in lying-in patients. Ineffectual urging to urinate in *newly married* women. Pressure upon bladder; feels as if it did not empty. *Sensation as if a drop of urine were rolling continuously along the channel*. Burning in urethra during micturition. Prostatic troubles; frequent urination, burning in urethra when not urinating. *[Thuja; Sabal; Ferr. pic.*] Urging and pain *after* urinating. Pain after lithotomy.

**Skin**.-Eczema of head, ears, face, and body; thick scabs, dry, and itch violently; *scratching changes location of itching*. Fig-warts pedunculated. [*Thuja*.] Arthritic nodes. Inflammation of phalanges. Night-sweats.

**Extremities**.-Muscles, especially of calves, feel bruised. *Backache; worse in morning before rising*. Extremities feel beaten and painful. Joints stiff. *Crural neuralgia*. Dull aching of nates extending to hip joint and small of back.

**Modalities**.-Worse, anger, indignation, grief, mortification, loss of fluids, onanism, sexual excesses, tobacco; least touch on affected parts. *Better*, after breakfast, warmth, rest at night.

**Relationship**.-Inimical-. *Ranunc. bulb*.
Complementary: *Caust.; Colocy*.
Compare: *Ferrum pyrophos*. (tarsal cysts); *Colocy.; Caust.; Ign.; Phos. ac.; Calad.* Antidote. *Camph*.

**Dose**.-Third to thirtieth potency.

## Colocynthis (Bitter Cucumber)

Often indicated in the transition season when the air is cold,
but the sun is still powerful enough to heat the blood.
Develops most of its symptoms in the abdomen and head, causing intense neuralgias. It is especially suitable for irritable persons easily angered, and ill effects therefrom. Women with copious menstruation, and of sedentary habits. Persons with a tendency to corpulency. The neuralgic pains are nearly always relieved by pressure. Cramps and twitching and shortening of muscles. Constrictions and contractions. Cysto-spasm following operations on orifices. [*Hyper.*] Urinous odor of perspiration.. *(Berb.; Nitr. ac.]* Agonizing pain in abdomen, causing patient to bend double, is most characteristic. Sensations: Cutting, twisting, grinding, contracting and bruised; *as if clamped with iron bands*.

**Mind**.-Extremely irritable. Becomes angry when questioned. Mortification caused by, offense. Anger, with indignation. [*Cham.; Bry.; Nux.*]

**Head**.-Vertigo when turning head *to the left*. Lateral cutting headache, with nausea, vomiting. Pains (better pressure and heat) with soreness of *scalp*. Burning pains, digging rending, and tearing. Frontal headache; worse, stooping, lying on back, and moving eyelids.

**Eyes**.-Pains sharp, boring, *better pressure*. Sensation on stooping, as if eye would fall out. Gouty affections of eyes. Violent pain in eyeballs which precede the development of glaucoma.

**Face**.-Tearing, shooting, and swelling of face; left side great soreness. Get relief from pressure. [*China*.] Neuralgia, *with chilliness;* teeth seems too long. *Sounds re-echo in ears.* Pain in stomach, always with pain of teeth or head.

**Stomach**.-Very *bitter* taste. Tongue rough, as from sand, and feels scalded. Canine hunger. Feeling in stomach as if something would not yield; drawing pain.

**Abdomen**.-Agonizing cutting pain in abdomen *causing patient to bend over double*, and pressing on the abdomen. Sensation as if stones were being ground together in the abdomen, and would burst. Intestines feel as if bruised. Colic with cramps in calves. Cutting in abdomen, especially after anger. Each paroxysm is attended with general agitation and a chill over the cheeks, ascending from the hypogastrium. Pain in small spot below navel. *Dysenteric stool renewed each time by the least food or drink. Jelly-like* stools. Musty odor. Distention.

**Female**.-*Boring pain in ovary. Must draw up double, with great restlessness.* Round, small cystic tumors in ovaries or broad ligaments. Wants abdomen supported by pressure. Bearing-down cramps, causing her to bend double. [*Opium*.]

**Urine**.-Intense burning along urethra during stool. Vesical catarrh, discharge like fresh white of egg. *Viscid. [Phos. acid]* fetid; small quantities, With frequent urging. Itching at orifice. Red, hard crystals, adhering firmly to vessel. Tenesmus of bladder. Pains on urinating *over whole abdomen*.

**Extremities**.-*Contraction of muscles.* All the limbs are drawn together. Pain in right deltoid. *[Guaco.] Cramp-like pain in hip*; lies on affected side; pain from hip to knee. Spontaneous luxation of the hip-joints. Stiffness of joints and shortening of tendons. Sciatic pain, left side, drawing, tearing; better, *pressure and heat;* worse, gentle touch. Contraction of the muscles. Pain down right thigh; muscles and tendons feel too short; numbness with pains. [*Gnaphal*.] Pain in left knee joint.

**Modalities**.-*Worse*, from anger and indignation. *Better,* doubling up, hard pressure, warmth, lying with head bent forward.

**Relationship**.-Antidote- *Coffea; Staphis.; Cham. Colocynth* is the best antidote to lead poisoning. (Royal).

Compare: *Lobelia erinus* (violent cork-screw-like pains in abdomen). *Dipodium punctatum* (*Writhing*. Twisting like a dying snake. Intractable insomnia.). *Dioscor.; Chamom.; Coccul.; - Merc.; Plum.; Magn. phos.*,

**Dose**.-Sixth to thirtieth

When you compare the emotional and bladder symptoms of these two remedies, *Staphysagria* is the correct remedy.

## A Word on Repertory Computer Programs

As seen above, Homeopathy is particularly suited to computers. Looking at the process of repertorization, it becomes immediately apparent that a machine could better do this time-consuming process. Once again, I must caution that the information retrieved is only as good as the information inputted in the first place.

Repertorization is the end of a long and sometimes tedious, process. Taking a case, and the analysis that follows, is the real core of any homeopathic process. Case analysis gives you the rubrics to be put into the computer, and the machine will do the nuts and bolts process of repertorizing. The computer will output a number of remedies that may possibly fit the case. It is up to the practitioner to read materia medica and find the most appropriate remedy.

There are two major repertory programs available. *MacRepertory*, and *The Radar System*. Both products contain an extensive repertory program and a library, and offer a number of different packages; from the very basic repertory program with a core library, to professional programs that include a number of other features, including veterinary programs, multi-media programs that look at the various remedies in depth, and other programs that help with different analysis strategies.

On their repertory side, both programs enable the Homeopath to take the case right on the computer, they have all the forms for case taking and will store the case as it would a regular patient file. Both libraries are extensive and contain not only modern books, but also some of the journals and case conferences, and writings of some of the original homeopaths.

As any Homeopath will tell you, you can never have enough books. To use either of these programs to their full potential would take hours of in-service, and lots of practice. They are very helpful tool, but only tools. For any of you who want to look at these computer programs, the information is in the back of the book. I would suggest you try both of them and figure out which program best suits you.

# Chapter IX

## Final Word

### Homeopathy *for* Nurses

I hope this book has stimulated your curiosity about Homeopathy and answered some basic questions. There certainly is a lot of information out there as you will see from the list of resources in the back of the book; and there are plenty of opportunities to learn more about this fascinating and effective therapeutic tool.

Because the practice of Homeopathy is not well regulated in the United States, many lay practitioners are getting into this field. It is my belief that Homeopathy, as a medical profession, should be practice by medical personnel. Nurses are the obvious choice to broaden the scope of homeopathic practice. Nurses have the scientific and medical background to be safe, effective practitioners in this field; as well as the theoretical basis to apply a holistic approach to healing.

The nature of Homeopathy and the realities of bedside nursing care are such that the application of Homeopathy in an "in-patient" setting would be difficult to say the least. Nevertheless, the knowledge of Homeopathy can be applied by Nurses as patient and family educators, counseling and helping to lead individuals to better health choices. Nurse practitioners, in particular, can integrate this discipline into their standard "out-patient" practice.

Today, information resources are more available then ever. If this book has peeked your interest in this amazing medical modality, I encourage you to go to some of the web sites listed in the resources; find topics that interest you, scout out the continuing educational opportunities, and take Homeopathy as far as you would like to.

# Appendix 1

## Resources

The following list of resources should be helpful when looking for more information about Homeopathy. The section is a list of homeopathic organizations. Their publications list seminars and other educational opportunities.

Homeopathic Nurses Association
4 Kellcourt Dr.
Atteboro, MA 02703
www.homeopathicnurses.org

Homeopathic Academy of Naturopathic Physicians
1412 W. Washington St.
Boise, ID 83702
208-336-3390
208-367-9242 (FAX)
www.bmathiew@spro.net

National Center for Homeopathy
801 N. Fairfax St., Suite 306
Alexandria, VA 22314
703-548-7790
703-548-7792 (FAX)
www.homeopathic.org

For other organizations go to the *Directory of Homeopathic Organizations* web site at:
www.extendedyears.com/lib/4010.html

## Schools of Homeopathy

New England School of Homeopathy
356 Middle St.
Amherst, MA 01002
413-256-5949
413-256-6223 (FAX)
www.nesh.com

The Canadian Academy of Homeopathy
1173 boul.du Mont-Royal
Outremont, QC Canada, H2V 2H6
514-279-6629
514-279-0111 (FAX)
www.homeopathy.ca

## Homeopathy Computer Programs

MacRepertory and Reference Works
1-877-937-5368
www.kenthomeopathic.com

Radar and Encyclopedia Homeopathica
Whole Health Now
1102 Pleasant St. PMB 816
Worcester, MA 01602
508-756-2987
508-767-1712
www.wholehealth.com

# *Appendix II*

## Glossary of Terms

**Acute disease:** In Homeopathy, self-limiting episode of illness in which the patient either recovers or dies.

**Aggravation**: An initial increase in symptoms when a remedy stimulates the action of the vital force.

**Allopathy:** The process of treating disease with medications that relieves symptoms by creating the opposite effect of that produced by the body in reacting to disease.

**Amelioration:** A decrease in the intensity of symptoms following an aggravation.

**Aphorism:** A brief statement of principle. In this case referring to the statements made by Dr. Hahnemann in *Organon of Medicine*, each of which are numbered.

**Chronic Disease:** In Homeopathic terms, a state of developed debility in which the vital force has been damaged so that it cannot regain health on its own.

**Centicimal Scale:** Homeopathic medication diluted one in one hundred.

**Concomitant Symptoms:** Those symptoms that occur at the same time but seldom have any kind of relationship except for time.

**Constitution:** A term that indicate individuals who react with the same or characteristic pattern of the vital force.

**Cure:** Permanent removal of the patient's symptoms and rebalance of the vital force.

**Decimal Scale:** Homeopathic medications diluted one to ten.

**Dosage:** In Homeopathy, the number of times the remedy is given.

**Exciting Cause:** A detrimental factor that produces disease in particularly sensitive people, so that weaknesses of the vital force are exposed.

**Homeopathy:** The practice of treating disease by giving medications able to produce the very symptoms that the disease processes elicit.

**Isopothay:** The practice of treating disease by giving the same substance that caused the symptom pattern.

**Key Note:** A characteristic symptom that identifies a remedy.

**Law of Similars:** *Similia Similibus curantur,* "Like cures like"

**Maintaining Cause:** The detrimental factor in the life of the individual that makes them more susceptible to ill health.

**Materia Medica:** A collection of symptom pictures of Homeopathic medication. A list of symptoms a remedy may produce and cure.

**Miasm:** A chronic or underlying affliction of the vital force from which it cannot recover on its own. In Homeopathy the three classic miasms are: Syphilitic, Sycotic and Psoric.

**Minimum Dose:** The smallest amount of medication required to stimulate the vital force to react.

**Modality:** Effects that change or define a symptom.

**Objective Symptoms:** Symptoms that we have observed through our senses.

**Nosode:** Remedies potentized from a disease product.

**Palliation:** The process by which symptoms are ameliorated without cure.

**Pollycrest:** Term used by Homeopathy to denote those remedies that are the most used and the best proven.

**Potency:** The number of times a Homeopathic medicine has been diluted and secussed.

**Potentization:** The process of making Homeopathic medications by serial dilutions and secussions.

**Predisposition:** The inherent weaknesses in the vital force that arise from miasms.

**Prescribing Symptoms:** The unusual or distinctive symptoms that characterize each patient and the manifestation of the illness.

**Presenting Symptoms:** The chief complaint of each patient.

**Prover:** A healthy person who takes a Homeopathic medication with the intent of proving it.

**Proving:** The process by which the properties of Homeopathic medications are found.

**Pseudo-Chronic Disease:** Originating from the maintaining cause and disappearing when that cause is removed.

**Remedy:** The name given to Homeopathic medications.

**Repertory:** A dictionary of symptoms produced by Homeopathic remedies.

**Rubric:** A class or category. In the case of Homeopathy it is the category of symptoms found in the Homeopathic Repertories.

**Samuel Hahnemann:** Father of Homeopathy and author of *Organon of Medicine*.

**Similimum:** The Homeopathic remedy that has produced a symptom picture most similar to that of the patient.

**Subjective Symptom:** The symptom experienced only by the patient.

**Secussion:** The process of vigorously shaking a solution of Homeopathic medications during its preparation between dilutions.

**Suppression:** The disappearance and reappearance of other symptoms in the opposite direction of the law of cure.

**Symptom:** A manifestation of discomfort or dis-ease that is abnormal for the patient.

**Symptom Picture:** A characteristic group of symptoms that is either applied to a patient condition or to the picture produced by a remedy.

**Total Symptom Picture:** Contains the entire symptom picture of the patient.

**Vital Force:** That process or energy that makes an organism alive rather than dead and corrects or maintains the organism within a set pattern.

**Vitality:** The energy available to sustain life.

# Appendix III

## Bibliography


Allen, Karen B. (1994). *A Tutorial and Workbook for the Homeopathic Repertory*. Homeopathic Tutorials. Redmond, WA.

Boericke, W. (1998). *Homeopathic Materia Medica and Repertory*. B Jain Publishers. London, England.

Clarke, John Henry. (1962). *A Dictionary of Practical Materia Medica*. Health Sciences Press. Sussex, England.

Hahnemann, Samuel. (1996). *The Organon of Medicine, First Inaugural English Translation of the Sixth Edition*. Cooper Publishing. Blaine, WA.

Kent, J.T. (1989). *Repertory of the Homeopathic Materia Medica*. 6th Ed. World Homeopathic Links. New Deli, India.

Morrison, Roger. (1993). *Desk Top Guide to Keynotes and Confirmatory Symptoms*. Hahnemann Clinic Publishing. Albany, CA.

Murphy, Robin. (1993). *Homeopathic Medical Repertory, a Modern Alphabetical Repertory*. 1st Ed. Hahnemann Academy of North America. Pagosa Springs, CO.

Murphy, Robin. (2000). *Homeopathic Remedy Guide*. 2nd Ed. . Hahnemann Academy of North America. Blacksburg, VA.

Rowe, Todd. (1998). *Homeopathic Methodology, Repertory, Case Taking and a Case Analysis, the Introductory Homeopathic Workbook*. North Atlantic Books. Berkley, CA.

Roy, Margaret. (1999). *The Principals of Homeopathic Philosophy, a Self-Directed Learning Text*. Winter Press. London, England.

Wright, Elizabeth. (1999). *A Brief Study Course in Homeopathy*, B Jain Publishers. New Deli, India.

# Appendix IV

## Index


*acute disease* 12, 41, 60, 61
*aggravation* 15, 16, 29, 30
*allopathic* 2, 11, 12, 14, 19, 45, 48, 50, 51, 55
*ameliorate* 29
*aphorism* 10, 20, 47, 51
*chronic disease* 12, 13, 50, 51
*concomitant symptoms* 34, 35, 52
*constitutional* 12, 45, 46, 55, 61
*cure* 6, 9, 14, 15, 16, 17, 31, 35, 36, 44, 51
*exciting cause* 12
*Law of Similars* 17
*materia medica* 6, 31, 39, 40, 41, 43, 44, 49, 57, 58
*miasm* 10, 13, 14
*miasmatic* 13, 14, 40
*minimum dose* 5, 20
*modality* 2, 52, 67
*nosodes* 40
*palliation* 15, 16
*polycrests* 39, 40, 46
*potency* 18, 19, 43, 57, 61, 64
*potentization* 18, 19
*predisposition* 11, 13
*prescribing symptoms* 34
*presenting symptoms* 34, 52
*prover* 6, 24, 29
*proving* 5, 6, 7, 20, 23, 24, 28, 29, 39, 40, 41, 57
*pseudo-chronic diseases* 13
*remedy* 5, 9, 16, 19, 24, 28, 31, 36, 39, 43 46, 50, 53, 57 63, 65
*repertory* 6, 23, 25, 27, 29, 41, 43, 56, 65
*rubric* 6, 7, 23, 27, 56, 58, 66
*Samuel Hahnemann* 1, 2, 5, 10, 12, 16, 18, 20, 23, 31, 43, 47, 51
*secussions* 18
*simillimum* 6
*suppression* 15, 16, 62
*symptom* 5,9, 12, 15, 18, 20, 23, 27, 30, 33, 36, 41, 50, 52, 58, 62
*vital force* 5, 9, 10, 11,18, 31, 33, 35, 39, 45
*vitality* 10, 13, 28, 30, 31, 44, 48, 52, 56